LECTURE NOTES ON RHEUMATOLOGY

Lecture Notes on Rheumatology

John Edmonds MB BS FRACP
Staff Physician, St George Hospital, Sydney, Australia

Graham Hughes MD FRCP
Consultant Rheumatologist, St Thomas' Hospital, London SE1

Blackwell Scientific Publications

OXFORD LONDON EDINBURGH

BOSTON PALO ALTO MELBOURNE

© 1985 by
Blackwell Scientific Publications
Editorial offices:
Osney Mead, Oxford, OX2 0EL
8 John Street, London, WC1N 2ES
23 Ainsdale Place, Edinburgh, EH3
  6AJ
52 Beacon Street, Boston
  Massachusetts 02108, USA
667 Lytton Avenue, Palo Alto
  California 94301, USA
107 Barry Street, Carlton
  Victoria 3053, Australia

First published 1985

Set by Butler & Tanner Ltd
Frome and London

DISTRIBUTORS

USA
  Blackwell Mosby Book Distributors
  11830 Westline Industrial Drive
  St Louis, Missouri 63141

Canada
  Blackwell Mosby Book Distributors
  120 Melford Drive, Scarborough
  Ontario M1B 2X4

Australia
  Blackwell Scientific Publications
    (Australia) Pty Ltd
  107 Barry Street
  Carlton, Victoria 3053

British Library
Cataloguing in Publication Data

Edmonds, J.
  Lecture notes on rheumatology.
  1. Rheumatism
  I. Title   II. Hughes, G. R. V.
  616.7′23   RC927

  ISBN 0-632-00368-5

Contents

Preface

It is perhaps surprising that it has taken so long to include a text on rheumatology in the Lecture Notes series. For the enthusiast, rheumatology has the attractions of combining a very 'clinical' subject with a rapidly broadening scientific base.

In this volume we have included new scientific concepts, but have not forgotten that rheumatology is a very practical, clinical and pragmatic subject.

We are grateful to our colleagues who have helped with comments, criticisms and illustrations, to our wives, Sue and Monica, who helped with the proof reading, and to Miss Penny Smart, who helped us through the final preparation of this book.

John Edmonds
Graham Hughes

1 Introduction

SCOPE OF RHEUMATOLOGY

Rheumatology is concerned with diseases of the joints and connective tissues. These structures can be damaged by a variety of pathological processes including infection, inflammation, degeneration, metabolic disturbances and systemic diseases such as leukaemia or haemochromatosis, which have their principal effect on other body systems.

The full list of disorders falling within the province of rheumatology is a long one and includes well over a hundred defined conditions. These notes concentrate on those which are common or are important because they require early recognition for correct management.

Until the aetiology of the various arthropathies is understood, attempts at classification are necessarily unsatisfactory. Table 1.1 is simply a list of the major groups of rheumatic diseases.

Table 1.1 Major groups of the rheumatic diseases

Group	Disease
Inflammatory arthritis of unknown aetiology	Rheumatoid arthritis Seronegative arthropathies: ankylosing spondylitis, Reiter's syndrome, psoriatic arthritis, enteropathic arthritis
Connective tissue disease	Systemic lupus erythematosus Scleroderma, progressive systemic sclerosis The arteritides: polyarteritis nodosa, other forms of arteritis Dermatomyositis and polymyositis Sjögren's syndrome
Crystal deposition disease	Gout Pseudogout Others

1

Table 1.1 *continued*

Group	Disease
Degenerative joint disease	Primary Secondary
Arthritis associated with infection	Septic arthritis Non-septic arthritis occurring in association with recognised infections: *bacterial*, e.g., gonococcus, meningococcus, salmonella, shigella; *viral*, e.g., rubella, hepatitis, mumps; *other*, e.g., fungal, protozoal etc. Post-infective arthritis: rheumatic fever, post-salmonella and shigella
Arthritis associated with systemic disease	Cardiovascular: bacterial endocarditis Endocrine: acromegaly, thyroid and parathyroid disease, diabetes Gastroenterological: inflammatory bowel disease, Whipple's disease Haemopoietic: haemophilia, haemoglobinopathies, leukaemia, myeloma Heritable developmental and storage diseases: Marfan syndrome, hypermobility syndrome Immunological: hypogammaglobulinaemia, serum sickness Metabolic: haemochromatosis, hyperlipoproteinaemia Metabolic bone diseases: osteoporosis, osteomalacia Neurological: neuropathic arthropathy Renal: chronic renal failure, chronic dialysis Respiratory: hypertrophic pulmonary osteoarthropathy Miscellaneous: sarcoidosis, amyloidosis
Non-articular rheumatism and localised pain	Tenosynovitis, bursitis, fibrositis Enthesophathies: tennis elbow Entrapment neuropathies: carpal tunnel syndrome Postural and post-traumatic syndromes Localised pain syndrome: shoulder pain, foot pain

It is included here to provide a brief summary of the main areas this book will cover and to draw attention to the range of disorders which cause arthritis. It is also useful to have a check list of disease subgroups such as this, particularly when confronted with the patient whose disease is atypical and does not fall clearly within one of the common diagnostic categories.

RHEUMATIC DISEASES IN PERSPECTIVE

It is obvious that, within the long list of rheumatic diseases, some are very common and others exceedingly rare. Some are uncommon but of importance because failure to recognise them early and treat them correctly may result in long-term deformity.

Commonest rheumatic diseases

Non-articular rheumatic syndromes—soft tissue rheumatism
Degenerative joint disease including spondylosis and disc disease
Rheumatoid arthritis
Gout
Systemic lupus erythematosus

Rheumatic diseases requiring early recognition and treatment

Septic arthritis
Juvenile chronic polyarthritis
Polymyalgia rheumatica with giant cell arteritis
Rheumatoid arthritis

2 Normal Joint Structure and Synovial Fluid

Joints are divided into three types:

1 Fibrous joints which allow almost no movement, e.g. cranial bone sutures.

2 Cartilaginous joints which allow limited movement, e.g. articulations between vertebral bodies, pubic symphysis.

3 Synovial joints which allow a wide range of free movement, e.g. all the joints of the limbs.

Only the synovial joint will be considered in more detail as it is this type which is usually involved in rheumatic disease. The intervertebral disc will be discussed in the section on degenerative disease.

SYNOVIAL JOINTS

Synovial joints (Fig. 2.1) have several characteristic features:
Opposing bony surfaces, covered with articular cartilage.

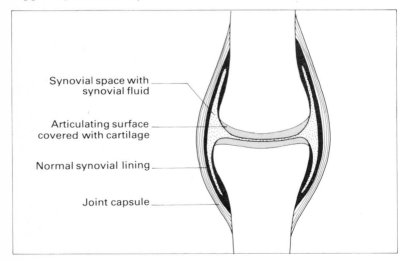

Synovial space with synovial fluid

Articulating surface covered with cartilage

Normal synovial lining

Joint capsule

Fig. 2.1 The synovial joint.

A joint cavity which is only a potential space in life.
A surrounding fibrous capsule.
A synovial membrane which lines the whole interior of the joint space with the exception of the articular cartilage.
Lubrication with synovial fluid.

Articular cartilage

Usually hyaline.
Firmly attached to underlying bone by its deep calcified layer.
Smooth surface without covering perichondrium.
Contains neither nerves nor blood vessels.
Derives nourishment from the vascular network of adjacent synovium, synovial fluid, blood vessels in the underlying bone.

Fibrous capsule

Consists of white fibrous tissue thickened in some areas to form named ligaments.
Usually attached to bone close to the edge of the articular surface.
Has little elasticity and causes pain if subjected to sustained tension.

Synovial membrane

Forms a relatively smooth lining surface covering all of the interior of the joint with the exception of articular cartilage and articular discs, or menisci. In some joints fringe-like processes (synovial villi) project into the joint cavity.
Consists of a layer of surface cells (synoviocytes) 1–3 cells deep overlying fibrous, fatty, or areolar connective tissue which contains the synovial blood vessels, capillary loops and lymphatics.
The membrane is capable of both phagocytic and synthetic activity and this correlates with the function of the two different types of synoviocytes recognised on electron microscopy:
— cell type A: appears to be responsible for removing particulate matter from the joint cavity and transferring it to cells in the deeper part of the membrane
— cell type B: synthesise and secrete the hyaluronate-protein complex of synovial fluid.
Is poorly supplied with nerve fibres and is relatively insensitive to pain.

SYNOVIAL FLUID

Viscous, pale yellow and clear. Present in small amounts (e.g. 0.1–4.0 ml in knee joint). Consists of a dialysate of plasma and hyaluronate-protein complex.

Constituents (Table 2.1)

1 Hyaluronate-protein complex.
— secreted by type B synoviocytes
— responsible for the fluid's high viscosity
— concentration is decreased in presence of inflammation.
Mucin clot test. Addition of acetic acid to synovial fluid precipitates the hyaluronate-protein complex as mucin. In normal fluid with high concentration of hyaluronate, the clot is tight, white and ropy; in inflammatory fluid, with a low concentration of hyaluronate, the clot is poor, fragmented or friable.
2 Proteins.
— normal concentration is about one-third of that in plasma (transudate) and is mainly albumin; there is no fibrinogen and the fluid does not clot
— in inflammatory fluid the protein concentration rises to approach that of plasma (exudate); fibrinogen enters the fluid which can then clot.
3 Other.
— electrolytes, uric acid, glucose, etc. present in approximately the same concentration as plasma

Table 2.1   Normal synovial fluid

Synovial fluid	Average value	Range
Volume (in knee) (ml)	2	0.1–4.0
Total protein (g/l)	20	10–30
Leucocytes/mm³	<200	30–200
Lymphocytes (%)	50	20–80
Mononuclear (%)	15	2–40
Polymorphs (%)	<25	10–60
Glucose ⎫ Uric acid ⎬ Electrolytes ⎭	Approximately the same as plasma	

— lysosomal enzymes present in very low concentration and correlate roughly with the cell count

— cells: total leucocyte count usually less than $150/mm^3$, predominantly lymphocytes with some monocytes and polymorphonuclear cells, also occasional synovial lining cells.

Functions

Lubricates the joint and supplies nutriment to avascular articular cartilage.

3 HLA Antigens and Rheumatic Diseases

The association between certain diseases and specific HLA antigens has been a major biological discovery because it provides an insight into the complex contribution of genetics and immunology to the pathogenesis of these diseases.

One of the earliest reported associations, and still the most striking, is that between ankylosing spondylitis and HLA-B27. The antigen B27 occurs in 6–10% of Caucasians but is present in more than 90% of patients with ankylosing spondylitis. Some of the other seronegative arthropathies also show increased frequency of B27 and, more recently, associations have been reported between other rheumatic diseases and antigens determined by other genes of the major histocompatibility complex. This chapter outlines the nature of the HLA system, the rheumatic disease associations with HLA antigens, and the pathogenic and clinical significance of these associations.

THE HLA SYSTEM

HLA Antigens

These are cell surface glycoproteins which are present on nucleated cells. Their function is not fully understood but they are the cellular markers of individuality and they have an important role in immunological reactivity at the level of cellular communication.

There are two main groups of antigens; the class I antigens (HLA-A, B and C) are found on most nucleated cells, the class II antigens (HLA-D/DR) are restricted to certain cells within the immune system.

The class I antigens have two components: a small fragment identified as $\beta2$ microglobulin, and a larger component which carries the antigenic specificity. The class II antigens also have two chains. The DRβ chain plays an important role in the functional expression of these antigens recognised as the HLA-D specificity. The base of the antigen is anchored in the cell membrane and the remainder projects above the cell surface with the antigenic portion exposed at the distal end.

Genetics of the HLA system

Although any one individual has a limited number of antigens on the cell surface—his or her pattern of biological individuality—the HLA system is strikingly polymorphic and a large number of different antigens have been identified. The HLA antigens are genetically determined and it is possible to divide the antigens into groups on the basis of the gene locus which codes for them.

These loci, on chromosome 6, have been designated A, B, C and D/DR (Fig. 3.1). At each locus, a number of different alleles (alternatives) may occur and these code for the antigens of the A, B, C, D/DR series. International studies have identified about 20 different antigens of the A locus, 30 antigens of the B locus, 8 of the C locus, about 10 of the D locus, and a similar number of the DR specificity.

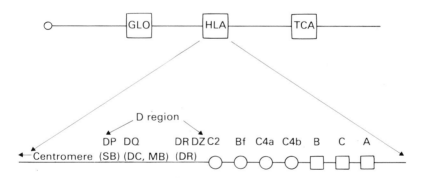

GLO = Glyoxylase
HLA = Human leucocyte antigen
TCA = T cell antigen

Fig. 3.1 Diagrammatic representation of the short arm of chromosome 6. Class I loci are located away from the centromere and code for HLA-A, B and C antigens.
Class II region is complex; it is located on the centromeric side of the MHC and codes for α and β chains of the HLA-D and DR antigens.
Class III loci lie between these regions and code for the complement components C2, Bf and C4.

Since the genes for HLA antigens are co-dominant and one allele occurs at each locus of the paired homologous chromosome, an individual will express two antigens determined at each locus. One chromosomal set, known as the haplotype, is inherited in a Mendelian manner from each parent (Fig. 3.2). An individual will

Haplotypes

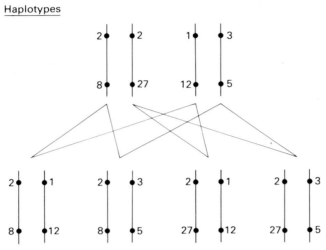

Fig. 3.2   HLA inheritance following Mendelian pattern.

therefore express two antigens of the HLA-A series (from the group of 20 possible), two antigens of the HLA-B series (from the group of 30 possible), and so on. If an individual is homozygous at one locus (carrying the same allele on each chromosome) only one antigen of that series will be detectable.

The chromosomal area coding for the HLA antigens is known as the major histocompatibility complex (MHC). The MHC also contains genes coding for complement components C2, C4 and Factor B and others which control a variety of functions, many of which are probably related to immunological reactivity.

Detection of HLA antigens

Antigens of the A, B, C and DR series are detected serologically using specific antisera and complement in a microlymphocytotoxicity test. Full tissue typing requires a large panel of specific antisera and is a complex and lengthy laboratory procedure.

Antigens of the D locus series were originally identified by the proliferative response of lymphocytes of non-compatible subjects when mixed together in tissue culture in a system known as mixed lymphocyte reaction. It was later found that specificities detectable serologically on B lymphocytes are similar to those expressed by the MLR and these have been termed the D-related (DR) antigens.

HLA nomenclature

This has been internationally standardised. Antigens are identified by the locus which codes for them: HLA-A1, HLA-A2, HLA-B5, HLA-B27, etc. Antigens which, on further international workshop testing, may be shown to contain more than one specificity are identified by the prefix 'w', e.g. HLA-Cw1, HLA-Dw5, etc.

Distribution within populations

The frequency of occurrence of HLA antigens varies between population groups. In some Caucasian populations frequencies are:

HLA-A1	16%	HLA-B5	6%
HLA-A2	28%	HLA-B7	10%
HLA-A3	14%	HLA-B8	10%
HLA-A29	4%	HLA-B12	14% etc.

In different racial groups, e.g., Japanese, American Indians, the frequencies of certain antigens may differ considerably.

When HLA antigens and disease associations are considered, the significance is determined by the frequency of the antigen in patients with the disease compared with the frequency of the antigen in the general population of the same racial origin.

ASSOCIATIONS BETWEEN HLA ANTIGENS AND RHEUMATIC DISEASE

The seronegative arthropathies show a strong association with HLA-B27. It has also become clear that rheumatoid arthritis shows a significant association with HLA-Dw4 and DR4. Some of the recognised associations are shown in Table 3.1.

HLA associations have been reported in a number of other

Table 3.1   HLA antigens and arthritis

Disease	HLA antigens	% Patients	% Controls
Ankylosing spondylitis	B27	90–95	6–10
Reiter's syndrome	B27	75–90	6–10
Psoriatic arthritis			
with peripheral arthritis	B27	10–20	6–10
with spondylitis	B27	50–60	6–10
Inflammatory bowel disease			
peripheral arthritis	B27	6–8	6–10
spondylitis	B27	50–60	6–10
Reactive arthritis			
Salmonella, Yersinia	B27	70–90	6–10
Rheumatoid arthritis	Dw4	35–55	10–20
	DR4	50–80	20–40

rheumatic diseases but in many the picture is confusing, either because of heterogeneity within the disease entity or as the result of changes which accompany the rapid and continuing developments in the HLA area particularly associated with the definition of HLA-D and DR specificities.

Juvenile chronic arthritis and systemic lupus erythematosus are examples of heterogeneous rheumatic diseases in which the true association of HLA antigens with certain subgroups is yet to be finally determined.

Significance of associations

PATHOGENETIC SIGNIFICANCE

The very strong association of HLA-B27 with ankylosing spondylitis and Reiter's syndrome must be relevant to the development of these disorders. Two main theories have been put forward to explain the association:

1   The antigen, because of its structure, acts as a receptor for or cross-reacts with an infectious agent and thus disturbs normal immunological and other functions.

2   The B locus allele HLA-B27 is strongly linked to another gene which permits the development of disease.

Which theory is correct has not yet been resolved and the mechanism underlying rheumatic disease associations with HLA-B27 may be quite different to that involved in HLA-D and DR associations. Answers to the questions posed by these recent findings will provide important insights into the pathogenesis of these rheumatic diseases and may lay the foundation for a preventative approach.

CLINICAL SIGNIFICANCE

Even in the case of the strongest HLA association—that of HLA-B27 in ankylosing spondylitis—the presence of the antigen cannot be used as a diagnostic test. Since B27 is present in 6–10% of the control population and ankylosing spondylitis occurs in no more than 20% of individuals with the antigen, the majority of those with HLA-B27 will be free of disease. Thus the 'false positivity' of HLA-B27 renders it unsatisfactory as a diagnostic investigation.

Clinical situations in which HLA-B27 may be useful include:
1   The patient with low back pain who lacks HLA-B27 is unlikely to have ankylosing spondylitis in the absence of psoriasis or inflammatory bowel disease.
2   The young patient with suggestive symptoms but inconclusive X-rays who is HLA-B27 positive should be followed up carefully.
3   The child, particularly a teenage boy, with lower limb pauciarticular arthritis who is HLA-B27 positive is more likely to follow the course of ankylosing spondylitis than that of typical juvenile chronic arthritis.

4 Clinical Approach to Diagnosis and Assessment

Patients with rheumatic diseases present with pain, aching or stiffness in joints, bones or muscles and/or joint swelling. There may be functional impairment or weakness with or without other symptoms and signs.

The clinician uses the history and physical examination to provide data for three basic steps in the clinical approach to diagnosis and assessment:

1 To determine the origin of the patient's symptoms, i.e. whether the patient has:
— arthritis (an arthropathy)
— non-articular or muscular pain
— another cause for the presenting symptoms.

2 To reach a diagnosis, i.e. determine the cause or category of the arthritis.

3 To assess disease severity, extent and treatment requirements in relation to the patient's general medical and social situation.

In rheumatology, most diagnoses are made clinically; investigations generally provide confirmation or help measure the extent of the disease process.

Origin of rheumatic pain

Is there evidence of an arthropathy?
Note:
— arthralgia means pain in a joint
— arthritis means joint inflammation but the word is commonly used in the broader sense to indicate the presence of joint pathology
— 'arthropathy' is possibly a better term to convey the idea of joint pathology without specifying inflammation but it is used less commonly.

Joint pain alone, arthralgia, is insufficient to confirm the presence of joint pathology.

Objective signs of arthritis or an arthropathy include:
— swelling
— tenderness
— limitation
— deformity
— crepitus
— heat and redness.

The combination of joint pain with one or more signs provides good evidence of joint pathology.

Diagnosis and differential diagnosis

Important information includes:
Patient's age and sex.
Characteristics of the arthritis:
— type: inflammatory, non-inflammatory
— duration: acute, chronic, intermittent
— extent: monoarthritis (one joint), oligoarthritis (2–4 joints), polyarthritis (more than 4 joints)
— distribution: joints involved. (peripheral, spine)
— pattern: large/small joints, upper/lower limbs, symmetry.
Additional features:
— systemic disease
— specific organ involvement: skin, bowel, eyes, etc.

Assessment

The assessment of disease severity, need and feasibility of treatment will include details of the patient's:
— functional capacity especially in relation to his or her social situation
— past and present treatment and its efficacy
— other medical conditions which may complicate the disease or its management
— social situation, responsibilities and expectations.

HISTORY AND PHYSICAL EXAMINATION

The history

The details of the history will vary considerably but certain basic points should always be covered.

1   Clarification of presenting symptoms.
Pain: site, duration, character, radiation, relieving and exacerbating factors; persistent or intermittent. Occasionally patients use a word such as pain, aching or soreness but in fact mean something else; it is vital to explore major symptoms to ensure mutual understanding.

Stiffness: severe and prolonged stiffness is an important feature of inflammatory arthritis. Both the duration and severity of morning stiffness are relevant.

To a rheumatologist, stiffness means the sensation of joint and/or muscular tightness and discomfort which wears off with activity; the term *gelling* is commonly used in the USA and is probably preferable.

Joint swelling: Has the patient observed joint swelling or other objective changes? Are they intermittent, persistent or progressive?

2   Extent of joint involvement.
Survey all joints: cervical spine, lower spine, temporomandibular joints, anterior chest wall, shoulders, elbows, etc., enquiring whether these joints have ever been involved, which are currently involved and which are causing most severe symptoms.

3   Profile of disease course.
Has the disease been progressive, intermittent, waxed and waned, shown long periods of remission or exacerbation? How often do flares occur and how long do they last?

4   Current status and functional effect.
What are the major current problems and which joints are most severely affected? To what extent is function limited; e.g. not at all, some activities difficult, some impossible, dependence on others? What ability is there to undertake personal functions, dress, prepare and eat food, maintain mobility?

5   Previous treatment and its effects.
Details should be as precise as possible, including:
Drug therapy: drugs used, their dose, effects and reason for termination.
Physical therapy: use of splints, exercises, physical aids, footwear and appliances.
Surgery: procedures, dates, surgeons and effects.
Details of other treatment should also be taken.

6   Extra-articular features.
These are common accompaniments to a variety of rheumatic diseases and often provide clues to diagnosis.

Relevant features: elbow nodules; skin rashes (psoriasis); eye involvement (dry eyes or iritis); inflammatory bowel disease; Raynaud's phenomenon; carpal tunnel syndrome and peripheral neuropathy; serositis and systemic disease (fevers, weight loss, etc.).
7   Past medical history.
It is always important to be aware of major past medical and surgical events. In patients with rheumatic disease it is particularly important to enquire about peptic ulcer disease and other gastrointestinal disturbances, asthma and allergies, previous adverse reactions to drugs and episodes of childhood arthritis.
8   Family history.
The disorders of particular importance include:
Metabolic disorders: haemophilia, haemochromatosis, chondrocalcinosis.
The seronegative spondarthropathies: enquire about severe back disease, uveitis, inflammatory bowel disease, psoriasis.
Other arthropathies: gout, rheumatoid arthritis, osteoarthritis, etc.
9   Social history.
During the process of taking the history it is essential to learn something about the patient and his or her response and attitude towards the disease. It is also necessary to know about the patient's domestic situation, occupation and responsibilities. Is the patient married and given support by the spouse? What is the effect of arthritis on occupation, occupational security, etc. Obtain a list of all current medications and drugs, both prescribed and proprietary (including alcohol and tobacco).

Physical examination

A full medical examination should always be performed; only the major and essential components of an examination of a patient with musculoskeletal complaints are outlined here.

GENERAL ASPECTS

General aspects of the musculoskeletal system examined include:
— body habitus
— posture: can the patient stand and is the posture normal?
— mobility: can the patient walk, are aids required, is there a limp, is gait normal?

JOINT EXAMINATION

The aim of a joint examination is to determine whether the joints are normal and if not, decide on the type of pathology affecting them, its extent and distribution. The examination includes two basic steps:

1   Look for:
— colour change of overlying skin
— muscle wasting
— joint swelling with joint deformity or malalignment
— range of active movement.

2   Feel for:
— swelling: is it soft tissue swelling or bony swelling?
— deformity: is the joint subluxed or dislocated?
— range of passive movement
— tenderness
— joint crepitus
— joint stability
— temperature change.

Axial and peripheral skeleton.   Examination should be systematic and include both the axial and peripheral skeleton. Information obtainable from joints heavily covered with muscle and ligaments, e.g. hips and spine, is less easily obtained than that of small peripheral joints. In some circumstances special manoeuvres yield additional information. Basically, however, at each joint or joint complex as much of the basic information should be obtained as possible.

a   Examination of axial skeleton includes:
— cervical spine
— lumbar spine: particularly range of movement
— chest expansion: to detect costovertebral joint involvement
— sternoclavicular joints
— manubriosternal joints
— temporomandibular joints.

b   Examination of the peripheral joints include:
— shoulders, elbows, wrists
— metacarpophalangeal, proximal interphalangeal and distal interphalangeal joints
— hips, knees
— ankle, subtalar and midtarsal
— metatarsophalangeal joints and the small joints of the toes.

NON-ARTICULAR FEATURES

Some of the more important non-articular features include:
— colour, particularly noting pallor
— elbow nodules
— nail pits and psoriasis
— sclerodactyly
— telangiectasia
— clubbing
— evidence of peripheral neuropathy
— endocrine abnormalities
— xerostomia and keratoconjunctivitis sicca
— rashes
— systemic features.

DIFFERENTIAL DIAGNOSES

The diagnosis is usually suggested once the nature and extent of the arthritis can be defined. By no means exhaustive, examples of the differential diagnoses suggested by common rheumatological situations include:

1 A hot, red, swollen joint, i.e. acute, severely inflammatory monoarthritis:
— infection
— crystal synovitis
— haemarthrosis
— seronegative arthritis (occasionally).

2 Acute monoarthritis:
— infection
— crystal synovitis
— trauma
— osteonecrosis
— onset of a chronic arthritis.

3 Chronic monoarthritis:
— chronic infection, e.g. tuberculosis
— internal derangement, trauma
— osteoarthritis (possibly secondary to trauma)
— seronegative arthritis
— rheumatoid arthritis.

4 Asymmetrical oligoarthritis:
— infection associated, e.g. gonococcal

— seronegative spondarthritis: psoriatic, Reiter's syndrome
— tophaceous gout.
5 Acute polyarthritis:
— infection associated, e.g. viral, septicaemic, post-infective
— allergic polyarthritis
— onset of a chronic polyarthritis.
6 Chronic polyarthritis:
— rheumatoid arthritis
— psoriatic arthritis
— primary generalised osteoarthritis
— a connective tissue disorder, e.g. systemic lupus erythematosus (S L E) etc.
7 Arthropathies suggested by certain non-articular features:
— fevers, weight loss, anorexia:
  infection associated arthropathies
  a connective tissue disorder
  inflammatory bowel disease
— skin disease:
  psoriasis: psoriatic arthritis
  facial rash: S L E, dermatomyositis
— eye disease:
  keratoconjunctivitis sicca: rheumatoid arthritis, connective tissue disease
    acute iritis: seronegative spondarthritis, sarcoidosis
    chronic iritis: juvenile chronic arthritis
    blindness: giant cell arteritis (G C A), polymyalgia rheumatica (P M R)
— clubbing:
  bacterial endocarditis
  hypertrophic osteoarthropathy
  pulmonary fibrosis
— Raynaud's phenomenon:
  progressive systemic sclerosis
  C R E S T₁ syndrome (*see* p. 159)
  mixed connective tissue disease (*see* chap. 13)
  other connective tissue disease
— proximal muscle weakness:
  dermato or polymyositis
  osteomalacia.

5 Laboratory Tests

Many new laboratory tests have been introduced in rheumatology during the past two decades, notably the various antinuclear antibodies, tests for immune complexes and tests for complement components. Although some, such as the Farr technique for anti-DNA antibodies, are highly specific diagnostically, it is still a fair generalisation that none solely contributes to patient management. Even the time-hallowed rheumatoid factor test has limited value in diagnosis and treatment.

RHEUMATOID FACTOR

Rheumatoid factors (RF) are antibodies directed against the Fc portion of altered gamma globulin. The routine laboratory tests for RF usually detect only IgM RF. By convention, therefore, *seropositive* and *seronegative* refer to the presence or absence of IgM antiglobulin in the serum. More recently, IgG RF (which is technically difficult to measure) has been found to be associated with vasculitis in rheumatoid arthritis (RA), and IgA RF with primary Sjögren's syndrome.

In addition to approximately 80% of patients with classical RA, IgM RF may be detected in a variety of conditions (*see* Chap. 6). Tests commonly used for RF are the latex fixation test and the sheep cell agglutination test.

Latex fixation tests

Human gammaglobulin is coated onto particles of polystyrene and a small volume of this suspension is added to 'doubling dilutions' of the test serum. Figure 5.1.

Sheep cell agglutination test (SCAT)

Instead of latex particles, sheep cells are used as the carrier for the gamma globulin. Sheep cells are coated with a 'subagglutin-

21

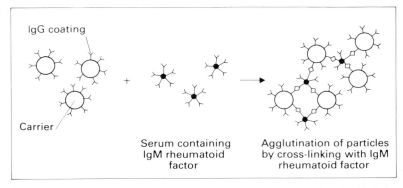

IgG coating

Carrier

Serum containing
IgM rheumatoid
factor

Agglutination of particles
by cross-linking with IgM
rheumatoid factor

Fig. 5.1   Rheumatoid factor method. The carrier used for the IgG is usually sheep RBCs (Rose Haaler test) or latex particles. Addition of serum positive for IgM RF causes visible agglutination of the particles.

ating' dilution of rabbit anti-sheep red cell IgG. These coated cells are then added to doubling dilutions of the patient's serum and the titre producing agglutination noted.

Occasionally sera contain heterophile antibody which will agglutinate normal sheep red cells, giving 'false positive' results. This problem is countered by first absorbing the test sera with sheep cells to absorb out the heterophile antibody.

ANTINUCLEAR ANTIBODY

Antibodies (of all classes) which react with constituents of the nucleus are found in a variety of conditions. They are traditionally measured by immunofluorescence.

Frozen tissue sections (usually rat liver) are incubated with the patient's serum. The sections are then washed, the antinuclear antibody (ANA), if present, adhering to the cell nuclei. The section is then incubated with fluorescent antisera to human gammaglobulin. This antiserum adheres to the patient's globulin at the sites where it is attached to the nuclei. These sites of antinuclear activity are detected by fluorescent microscopy (Fig. 5.2).

A variety of patterns may be observed:
— homogeneous, the commonest pattern especially in S L E and drug induced L E
— speckled, prominent in patients with mixed connective tissue disease
— nucleolar, rare, sometimes seen in scleroderma.
More recently, other methods such as counterimmunoelectropho-

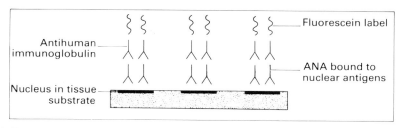

Fig. 5.2 Immunoflourescent ANA method. Frozen sections containing nuclei (usually rat liver) are prepared on slides. The test serum is added. Ig anti-nuclear antibody is present, this adheres to the nuclei and is then detected by the use of fluorescein-labelled anti-human Ig.

resis (C I E) and immuno-blotting have allowed much more detailed identification and even chemical definition of some of the antinuclear and anticytoplasmic antibodies. Though their clinical significance is still being evaluated, they are of sufficient importance to be listed (Table 5.1).

Table 5.1 Antinuclear and anticytoplasmic antibodies with antigens chemically characterised and incompletely characterised.

Antigens	Comment
Chemically characterised	
Double stranded D N A	S L E. Highly specific
Single stranded D N A	Non-specific
R N A	—
Histones	Some cases of drug L E
Jo-l	Polymyositis with pulmonary fibrosis
Incompletely characterised	
Ribonucleoprotein (R N P)	M C T D (high titres), S L E low titre
Ro (S S A)	Predominantly cytoplasmic. A N A-negative lupus. Sjögren's. Congenital heart block mothers
La (S S B)	Sjögren's. S L E
Sm	20% of S L E sera
R A P	Seropositive R A
Scl 70	Scleroderma
Centromere	C R E S T syndrome
Others	Over 20 precipitin systems now recognised. Clinical association not yet clear

Anti-DNA antibodies

Since their introduction into clinical practice in the late 1960s, anti-DNA antibodies have proved remarkably disease specific for SLE. Raised titres of anti-DNA antibodies are only rarely found in diseases other than SLE; very high titres are almost pathognomonic of the disease.

Anti-DNA antibodies are usually measured either by a sensitive immunoassay, e.g. the Farr technique; or by an immunofluorescent slide test. With the former test radioactive double stranded DNA is added to the test serum and any complexes formed are precipitated by ammonium sulphate (Fig. 5.3). The

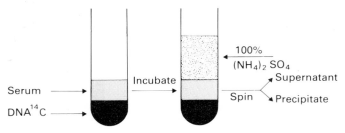

Fig. 5.3   Farr technique. ^{14}C-labelled DNA is added to test serum. DNA–anti-DNA complexes if formed, are precipitated on addition of 100% saturated ammonium sulphate. The amount of radioactivity in the precipitate portion thus measures the anti-DNA antibody activity of the serum (Hughes G.R.V., Cohen S.A., Lightfoot R.W., Meltzer J.T. & Christian C.L. (1971) The release of DNA into serum and synovial fluid. *Arthritis and Rheumatisim*, **14**, 259.)

immunoflourescence method makes use of the observation that the kinetoplast of the trypanosome *Crithidia* consists almost entirely of double stranded DNA. It is cheaper to perform, but less precise than the Farr technique.

Extractable nuclear antigens

For the detection of extractable nuclear antigens CIE is used. An extract of nuclear-rich tissue (conventionally calf thymus or rabbit spleen), after appropriate treatment, is placed in an agarose well, and test sera are placed in adjacent wells. When a current is applied across the agarose, precipitin reactions may be seen. By comparison with 'known' sera, the identity of these precipitating antibodies is found. There are at the present time over 20 such antinuclear and anticytoplasmic antibodies, of which a small number have some clinical significance.

RNP

Anti-RNP antibodies are seen in a small number of patients with severe Raynaud's phenomenon and ('sausage fingers') and arthritis—so called 'mixed connective tissue disease' (*see* p. 158). Although low titres of anti-RNP antibodies are also found in SLE, it is significant that in MCTD, the antibody is usually found in high titres and in the absence of other antibodies.

ANTI-RO (ANTI-SSA)

The Ro antigen is predominantly cytoplasmic. Hence occasional patients with anti-Ro antibodies may prove 'ANA-negative' on conventional testing. At the present time, the presence of Ro has been associated with a number of features:
— photosensitive skin rashes
— a tendency to thrombocytopenia
— Sjögren's syndrome
— rarity of renal disease
— an isolated finding in some mothers of children with congenital heart block.

ANTI-Sm

Found in a small number of SLE patients, and rarely in other conditions, the clinical significance of anti-Sm is unknown.

RAP

Rheumatoid arthritis precipitin (RAP), is also called anti-rheumatoid arthritis nuclear antigen (RANA). This antibody appears after infection with Epstein-Barr virus. It occurs in over 80% of RA patients.

JO-1

A number of precipitin systems are found in polymyositis. Anti-Jo-1, found in approximately 25% of polymyositis patients, may be associated with overlap features such as Raynaud's and pulmonary fibrosis. The antigen has been identified as histidyl t-RNA synthetase.

ANTI-CENTROMERE

This interesting antibody, anti-centromere, is directed against the centromere of dividing chromosomes and is not detected by conventional ANA methods. It appears to be associated with the CREST variant of scleroderma.

ACUTE PHASE REACTANTS

The ESR is still the most widely used test for acute phase reactivity in SLE, though measurements of blood and serum viscosity are preferred in some centres.

C-REACTIVE PROTEIN

This acute phase protein, C-reactive protein (CRP), made in the liver, has recently re-emerged as a useful test in rheumatology. In SLE (and in primary Sjögren's syndrome) patients appear unable to achieve high CRP levels, even when the disease is active and the ESR is well over 100. In infection, however, the CRP level *does* rise, though rarely to the levels seen in other conditions. This observation has some value both in contributing to a diagnosis of SLE, and (to a lesser extent) in the assessment of the SLE patient with fever.

SERUM AMYLOID-A PROTEIN

Serum amyloid-A (SAA) is the putative precursor of amyloid-A protein which forms the fibrils in secondary amyloidosis. As with CRP, elevation of SAA are modest in SLE, but high in RA and Still's disease. It is not yet known whether prolonged high levels of SAA foretell the development of amyloid.

COMPLEMENT

TOTAL HAEMOLYTIC COMPLEMENT (CH$_{50}$)

The end result of the complement cascade can be detected by the haemolysis of red blood cells. Because components of complement are also acute phase reactants, raised complement levels are found in many of the inflammatory rheumatic diseases, e.g. RA.

The fixation of complement by circulating immune complexes may result in low CH_{50} values, especially in SLE. Measurement of complement is clinically useful in SLE, where low values generally indicate active disease (though *not* necessarily renal disease) and in the synovial fluid, where, for example, low levels are seen in RA and high levels in Reiter's syndrome.

In the management of SLE, a rapidly falling CH_{50} level is one of the best warning signs of worsening disease.

COMPLEMENT COMPONENTS

Genetic deficiencies of all complement components (Clq, Clr, Cls, C2-9) occasionally occur and are associated with the tendency either to infection or to the development of connective tissue diseases. About half of those with C2 deficiency have autoimmune diseases, especially lupus.

In clinical practice, assays for C3 and C4 are carried out in most routine laboratories. Low C4 levels in SLE generally reflect disease activity.

IMMUNE COMPLEXES

There are well over 40 methods for the detection of immune complexes (IC). Each test depends on separate structural or functional characteristics of the immune complex. Thus different results are obtained by different tests in different diseases. Some generalisations are:

1   Circulating immune complexes (IC) are found in most of the connective tissue diseases.
2   IC are found in high titre in RA synovial fluid.
3   Very high levels of circulating IC are frequently associated with vasculitis.
4   The titre of circulating IC in any individual disease, e.g. SLE broadly reflects disease activity.
5   High titres of IC may also result, in part, from impaired clearance by the reticuloendothelial system.

The most commonly used method for the detection of IC is the Clq binding test, which depends on the property of certain IC to adhere to the first component of complement.

CRYOGLOBULINS

One of the simplest, and most often neglected, tests in rheumatology is cryoprecipitation. Blood is taken and allowed to clot at 37°C. The serum is kept at 4°C for 72 hours. The cryoprecipitate is washed and analysed for protein content. Polyclonal cryoprecipitates are seen in SLE, RA (especially with Sjögren's, Felty's and vasculitis) and some vasculitides.

SYNOVIAL FLUID ANALYSIS

Analysis of synovial fluid is mandatory in acute monoarthritis, and useful in patients with polyarthritis. Although there are many aspects to synovial fluid analysis the two main reasons for aspiration are culture and examination for crystals.

Synovial fluid examination may be diagnostic in septic arthritis and crystal deposition disease. In some cases, simple analysis of synovial fluid, based on its colour, clarity, viscosity and white cell count (WCC) allows a useful classification of the fluid changes into 4 'non-specific' categories (Table 5.2).

Table 5.2 Simple analysis of synovial fluid

Description	Normal	Non-inflammatory	Inflammatory	Septic
Colour	Colourless-straw	Straw-yellow	Off-white-yellow	Variable
Clarity	Clear	Clear	Translucent-opaque	Opaque-turbid
Viscosity	High	High	Low	Variable
WCC				
No. mm^3	<200	200–2000	3000–75 000	>50 000
% PMNL	<25	<25	>50	>90

Synovial fluid complement estimation (discussed previously) while theoretically of considerable diagnostic value in early polyarthritis, has not become widely used, possibly because of the technical difficulties involved.

Detailed discussion of synovial fluid crystal analysis is given in Chapter 18.

6 Rheumatoid Arthritis: Pathology and Pathogenesis

Rheumatoid arthritis (RA) is a chronic inflammatory disease which primarily affects synovium. Since the aetiology is unknown and there are no specific tests, the diagnosis is essentially clinical. It is unlikely to be an entirely homogeneous form of arthritis.

PATHOLOGY

Articular

MICROSCOPIC CHANGES

The synovial membrane is initially affected. Normal synovium is composed of a surface layer of synovicytes about two cell layers deep and underlying connective tissue stroma. In rheumatoid arthritis the main features are oedema and increased vascularity, proliferation of cells of the surface layer and infiltration of the stroma with lymphocytes and plasma cells (Fig. 6.1). The lymphocytes may aggregate into follicles (Fig. 6.2). There is also hypertrophy of synovial villi, accumulation of fibrin on the synovial surface and formation of pannus, which is granulation tissue growing across the surface of the articular cartilage from the adjacent synovium.

MACROSCOPIC CHANGES (Fig. 6.3)

Normal joint. The articulating surfaces are covered with cartilage. The remainder of the joint interior is lined with synovium.
Early diseases. Inflamed synovium and the effusion into the joint space cause joint swelling. Wasting of muscles around the joint is an important, early sequel.
Later features. The inflammatory effusion, in which the predominant cell is the polymorphonuclear leucocyte, contains high levels of lysosomal and other enzymes capable of degrading cartilage and leading ultimately to cartilage thinning. Later, pannus

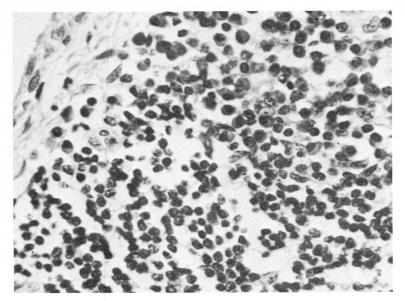

Fig. 6.1 Synovium in active R A, showing predominantly plasma cell (top) and lymphocyte infiltration. (H & E × 520) (Dr Shirley Amin, University Hospital of the West Indies.)

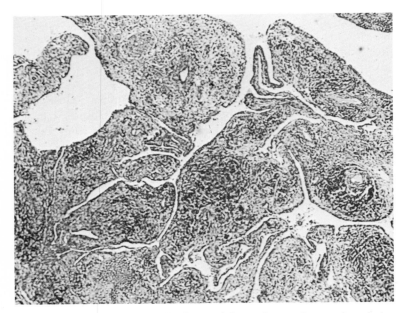

Fig. 6.2 Hypertrophied villi of synovial membrane due to chronic inflammation with lymphoid follicle formation. (H & E × 54) (Dr Shirley Amin, University Hospital of the West Indies.)

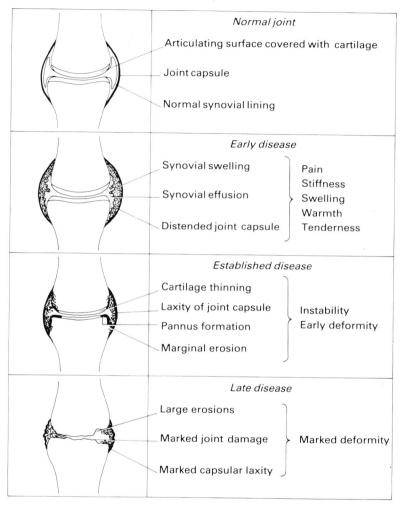

Fig. 6.3   Macroscopic changes in RA.

invades and grows across the cartilage. The pannus erodes cartilage and eventually invades bone to produce marginal erosions. Longstanding inflammation and effusion distend the joint capsule causing ligamentous laxity: the combined effects of joint damage, muscle wasting, instability and continued use lead ultimately to deformity.

Inactive disease.   After a variable period, synovial inflammation may become quiescent either spontaneously or as a result of treatment. If little structural damage has occurred, the joint may appear clinically and radiologically normal. If the joint has been damaged during the period of active inflammation, deformities will persist and may worsen as secondary degenerative changes ensue.

Non-articular

NODULES

The histology of the rheumatoid nodule provides the most diagnostically helpful pathology in RA since the nodule structure, although not pathognomonic, is remarkably consistent (Fig. 6.4). There are three distinct zones:
— inner area of necrotic material including fibrin, surrounded by
— palisade of radially arranged histiocytes and fibroblasts
— outer zone of chronic inflammatory cells: lymphocytes and plasma cells, and some fibroblasts.

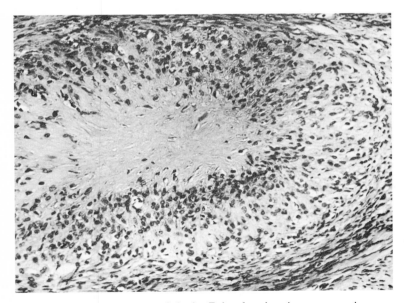

Fig. 6.4 Subcutaneous nodule in RA, showing inner necrotic zone, surrounding palisades of mononuclear inflammatory cells and an outer layer of chronic inflammatory cells and fibroblasts. (H & E × 160) (Dr Shirley Amin, University Hospital of the West Indies.)

OTHER NON-ARTICULAR FEATURES

Many of the non-articular features are due either to nodule formation or vasculitis, usually affecting small vessels.

AETIOLOGY

The aetiology of RA is unknown. The increased prevalence of RA in women and the tendency for disease to become quiescent during pregnancy implicate hormonal factors. There is also good evidence that immunological mechanisms are important.

Infective agents. An infective agent seems a likely exogenous stimulus although none has yet been incriminated. At present, attention is being directed to the possible role of various viruses.

Genetic factors. Patients with RA have been found to possess the HLA antigens Dw4 and DRw4 significantly more frequently than unaffected individuals.

Immunological factors. Immunological factors are considered to be of pathogenetic significance because:

— the presence of rheumatoid factors (RF) in the blood and synovial fluid shows a broad correlation with disease severity and the range of extra-articular features
— the synovial membrane shows many of the characteristics of an immunologically stimulated lymphoid organ.

Before outlining the proposed sequence of events leading to inflammation and tissue damage, it is useful to discuss the nature and significance of rheumatoid factor.

Rheumatoid factor (Fig. 6.5)

The precise mechanism of RF production is unknown. The appearance of RF during some chronic infections suggests that persistent immune stimulation provokes an antiglobulin response to complexed IgG.

DETECTION

The various tests for RF are detailed in Chapter 5.

IgM as antibody

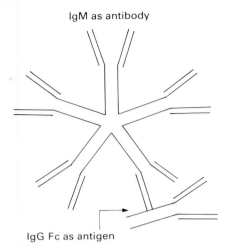

IgG Fc as antigen

Fig. 6.5   Rheumatoid factor. While rheumatoid factors (anti-IgG anti-bodies) may be of all immunoglobulin classes, the method commonly used—precipitation—only measures IgM RF.

CLINICAL SIGNIFICANCE

RF is not specific to RA. Some of the diseases in which RF are found are listed in Table 6.1. In RA, patients with RF are said to be 'seropositive'. The titre of RF is significant; high titres show a broad correlation with more severe disease and parti-cularly with some systemic manifestations, such as: nodules, vas-culitis, Sjögren's syndrome, peripheral neuropathy, lung involve-ment, and Felty's syndrome.

IgG and IgA RF are also found in 'seronegative' RA and in other types of inflammatory arthritis, such as ankylosing spon-dylitis, psoriatic arthritis, and juvenile chronic arthritis.

PATHOGENETIC SIGNIFICANCE

The role of IgM RF is not entirely clear. There is evidence that it is capable of fixing complement and it may facilitate the phag-ocytosis of immune complexes by polymorphs in the synovial fluid. Although its presence is strongly associated with a number of systemic manifestations of RA, it is unlikely to be the aetio-logical factor directly responsible for these.

IgG RF may have a more significant role in immune complex

Table 6.1   Diseases sometimes associated with rheumatoid factor

Group	Diseases/Subject
Connective tissue disease	Rheumatoid arthritis Sjögren's syndrome SLE Scleroderma Mixed connective tissue disease
Other diseases with immunological features	Chronic active hepatitis and other chronic liver disease Fibrosing alveolitis Paraproteinaemia Cryoproteinaemia
Chronic infections	Subacute bacterial endocarditis Pulmonary TB Infectious mononucleosis Syphilis Leprosy
Others	Normal older individuals Relatives of RA patients

activity within the joint, since it is responsible for a major portion of complement fixation and activation.

PATHOGENESIS

Although the factors responsible for initiating RA and for maintaining its chronicity are not understood, much is known about events within the synovial fluid and the synovial membrane and about the relationship between immunological and biochemical mechanisms of tissue damage.

SYNOVIAL COMPARTMENT ABNORMALITIES

The cell population and immunological environment of synovial fluid differ considerably from that within the synovial membrane. In active RA, the synovial fluid contains numerous polymorphonuclear leucocytes, there are high levels of immune complexes and evidence of complement activation. By contrast, the synovial membrane contains mononuclear cells and fibroblast-like cells and generates lymphokines, monokines and immunoglobulin, much of which has R F activity.

Recent studies on the microenvironment of the synovial membrane have shown the presence of macrophage-like cells, which strongly express HLA-DR antigens and are surrounded by T cells of the 'helper' type together with B cells and plasma cells. T cells of the 'suppressor' type are scarce and scattered. This suggests that the principal defect within the synovium lies with the lack of adequate T suppressor activity. As a result, B cell differentiation is promoted by the 'helper' cells and the DR+ macrophage-type cell may be the chief accessory involved in their antigenic stimulation.

MECHANISMS OF TISSUE DAMAGE

The immunological events within the synovium have two important results: there is an inflammatory response mediated by immune complexes and tissue destruction mediated by monokine stimulation of synovial cells.

Inflammatory response.   Rheumatoid factors and other immunoglobulins generated by the synovium are released into the synovial fluid and form immune complexes. IgG RF acts both as an antigen and antibody and is self-aggregating. Rheumatoid factors can fix complement and activation of the complement sequence is one stimulus to the attraction of polymorphs which clear immune complexes by phagocytosis. There are two locally harmful consequences of neutrophil phagocytic activity: first, the cell surface responds by a burst of oxidative metabolism which transforms molecular oxygen into highly reactive and damaging oxygen-derived free radicals, superoxide, hydroxyl ions and hydrogen peroxide; second, attempts to phagocytose large particles may result in the release of neutral proteases from the phagolysosomes. Thus rheumatoid factors and other locally generated immunoglobulins provoke an inflammatory response through extravascular immune complex mediated mechanisms.

Tissue damage.   It is now apparent that there are clear links between immunologically active cells such as lymphocytes and macrophages and the generation of prostaglandins and proteolytic enzymes which can break down collagen, cartilage and bone.

Cells of the monocyte-macrophage series, aided by lymphocytes, release a monokine (interleukin-1) which stimulates fibroblast-like cells in the synovium to secrete prostaglandin and proteases such as collagenase and proteoglycanase. Other factors released by the inflamed synovium lead to resorption of cartilage matrix by chondrocytes and the production of plasminogen activator.

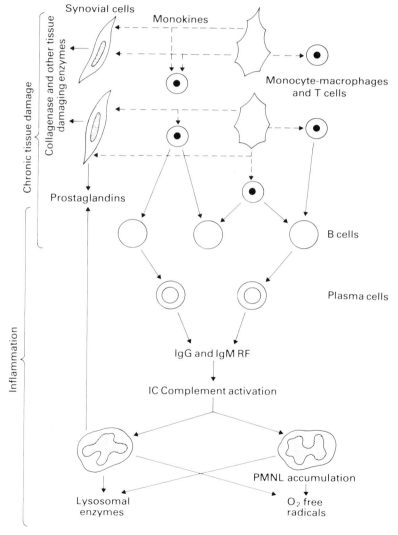

Fig. 6.6 Rheumatoid pathogenesis.

Thus, the interaction between the immunological invader cells and the local residents of synovium, cartilage and bone generate prostaglandins, and proteolytic enzymes, the mediators of continuing inflammation and tissue damage.

A schematic representation of the possible sequence linking defective immunoregulation, uncontrolled by appropriate synovial suppressor T cells, with immune complex mediated inflammation and monokine stimulated generation of tissue damaging enzymes is shown in Figure 6.6.

7 Rheumatoid Arthritis: Clinical Features

EPIDEMIOLOGY

Prevalence. About 1% of the adult population are affected but racial and geographical variation exists.

Distribution. The disease occurs world wide and prevalence is not influenced by climate.

Sex. The female:male ratio is 3:1.

Age. Childhood to old age. In patients under 16 years of age, the disease is termed juvenile chronic arthritis, discussed in Chapter 11. Peak age of onset is 35–55 years.

ONSET

Joint distribution

Polyarticular onset in about 80%; usually PIP, MCP, MTP joints and wrists. Mono-articular onset in about 20%; usually knee or wrist.

Mode of onset

Insidious in the majority; constitutional symptoms of fatigue and malaise may precede the arthritis by several months.

Explosive onset occasionally; it is usually polyarticular and may be accompanied by marked constitutional features.

Episodic in a minority with periods of arthritis alternating with phases of remission.

Palindromic onset is rare. Acute episodes of joint pain and swelling, usually affecting only one joint and lasting hours to days have been termed 'palindromic' rheumatism. About one-third of patients with palindromic rheumatism progress to RA while some develop SLE or another inflammatory joint disease.

SYMPTOMS

Stiffness, particularly after inactivity, is the hallmark of inflammatory arthritis; it is often severe, generalised and prolonged. In the mornings, it usually lasts for at least 20–30 minutes and may persist for several hours. Joint stiffness, without significant pain or swelling, may be the first symptom of inflammatory arthritis.

Pain, tenderness, swelling and limitation of movement of joints; oedema of the hands, ankles or feet may be prominent.

Functional impairment, with loss of grip strength, muscle power or mobility occurs early, particularly in polyarticular disease. Loss of hand power and grip may be prominent even when there is little evident synovitis.

Constitutional symptoms of malaise, tiredness, easy fatiguability and depression are common; anorexia and weight loss are less frequent and fever is rare.

Carpal tunnel syndrome occurs in up to 50% of patients with early disease.

SIGNS

In early disease:
Soft tissue swelling of joints due to synovial inflammation and effusion.

Tenderness.

Limitation of movement.

Warmth of affected joints.

Local oedema, particularly of the ankles; slight erythema may occur.

Muscle wasting occurs early around involved joints.

Note
1 While symmetrical joint involvement is usual, asymmetry of involvement may be present in early disease, particularly when the large joints are initially affected.
2 Hot, red joints are *not* a feature of RA but suggest either septic arthritis or crystal synovitis.
3 Fixed deformities are absent in early disease.
4 In some patients, particularly older males, the constitutional features may predominate, producing a clinical picture resembling neoplasia or infection.

In established disease:
Joint involvement is usually symmetrical.
Deformities are often present (see below).
Swelling may be due to persisting synovitis with synovial thickening and effusion, bony swelling of secondary degenerative changes or a combination of these.
Muscle wasting and weakness become more prominent.
Non-articular manifestations (*see* p. 46).

SPECIFIC ARTICULAR MANIFESTATIONS

The approximate frequency of individual joint involvement is shown in Fig. 7.1. Almost every synovial joint in the body may become involved in RA. The special characteristics of involvement of some joints are detailed below.

Hands

In early disease:
Muscle wasting.
MCP joint swelling with filling in of the hollows between the metacarpal heads when the fingers are flexed.
PIP joint swelling producing 'spindling'.
Tenosynovitis: flexor tendon synovitis which may impair function or cause finger triggering and dorsal sheath effusion.
DIP joint involvement is rare but may occur when all of the other hand joints are affected.

In later disease:
Subluxation of MCP joints; ulnar deviation of the fingers at the MCP level.
Button-hole deformity of fingers.
Swan-neck deformity of fingers.
Z deformity of the thumb, causing loss of pinch grip.
Tendon lesions: tendon attenuation with weakness may progress to tendon rupture causing finger drop.
These deformities should be noted and their effect on function assessed; this can be done quickly by measuring grip strength, pinch ability and the 'flexor deficit' of the fingers—the distance between the finger tip and palm when the patient attempts to clench the fist.

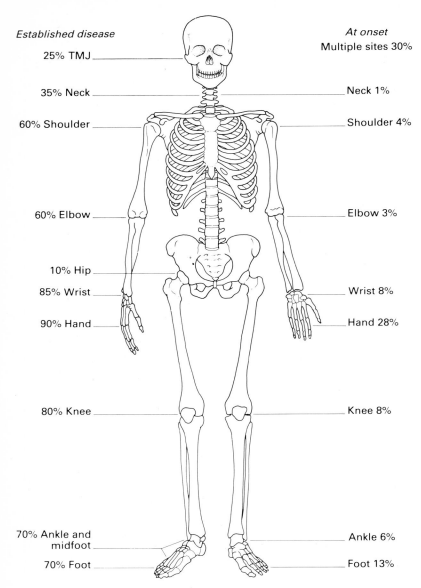

Established disease

25% TMJ

35% Neck

60% Shoulder

60% Elbow

10% Hip

85% Wrist

90% Hand

80% Knee

70% Ankle and
    midfoot

70% Foot

At onset

Multiple sites 30%

Neck 1%

Shoulder 4%

Elbow 3%

Wrist 8%

Hand 28%

Knee 8%

Ankle 6%

Foot 13%

Fig. 7.1 Frequency of joint involvement: at onset and in established disease.

Wrists

Ulnar styloid prominence and tenderness. Synovitis and erosion around the ulnar styloid may contribute to rupture or attenuation of the 4th and 5th extensor tendons (Fig. 7.2).
Subluxation.
Deviation of the hand to the radial or ulnar side.
Carpal tunnel syndrome caused by wrist and flexor tendon synovitis.

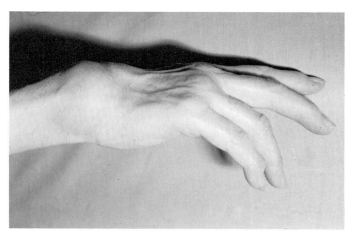

Fig. 7.2 Rupture of extensor tendons of 4th and 5th fingers with wrist synovitis subluxation.

Feet

MTP joint synovitis causes pain and tenderness across the ball of the foot—an early, common and severe feature.
MTP joint subluxation is common and causes callus formation over the tender, prominent metatarsal heads (Fig. 7.3).
Hallux valgus often with an overlying callus and bursal reaction (bunion).
Clawed toes.
Valgus deformity of mid and hind foot with flattening of the arch.
   The MTP joint is frequently an early site of radiological erosion.

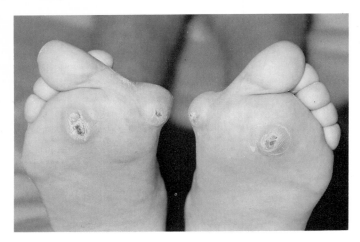

Fig. 7.3   MTP joint involvement with calluses.

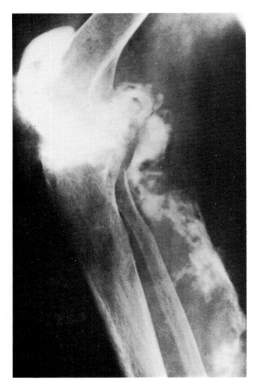

Fig. 7.4   Arthrogram showing rupture of the synovial sac posteriorly and tracking of contrast medium into the calf.

Knees

Quadriceps muscle wasting.

Baker's cyst: a synovial outpouching into the popliteal fossa associated with high intra-articular pressure which is often more easily seen than felt. Rupture of the cyst, with leakage of synovial fluid into the calf muscles, produces severe pain, swelling, tenderness and a positive Homan's sign which closely mimics a deep vein thrombosis.

The cyst and rupture of the cyst are readily diagnosed by arthrography—an X-ray after injection of radio-opaque contrast into the synovial cavity (Fig. 7.4).

Flexion deformity.

Lateral angular deviation in advanced disease.

Cervical spine

Atlanto-axial subluxation. Normally, the odontoid process of the axis is held firmly against the anterior arch of the atlas by the transverse ligament of the atlas. In RA, local synovitis causes slackening of the ligament, allowing the skull and the atlas to sublux forward during flexion; even more dangerous, the odontoid peg may be progressively eroded.

Subluxation is best detected on X-ray, when a lateral view of the neck in flexion will demonstrate a separation of the odontoid process from the arch of the atlas, exceeding 3 mm (Fig. 7.5).

Other changes: There is subluxation of one vertebral body on another; narrowing of disc spaces without significant osteophyte formation and erosion of apophyseal joints and vertebral bodies.

Note:

1   Cervical involvement may cause neck and occipital pain, vertebro-basilar insufficiency, and cervical myelopathy with long tract signs (uncommon).

2   All rheumatoid patients requiring a general anaesthetic should have a pre-operative X-ray of the cervical spine in flexion.

Other joints

Crico-arytenoid involvement may cause hoarseness and dyspnoea. Temporomandibular joint involvement may be a prominent, early feature.

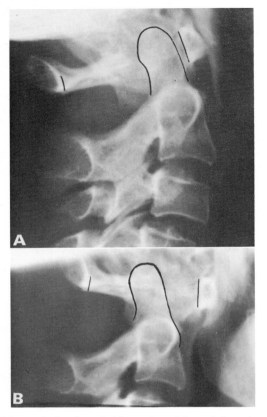

Fig. 7.5 RA cervical spine. **A** Normal position of the odontoid peg in extension. **B** Wide separation of the odontoid on full flexion of the neck.

NON-ARTICULAR MANIFESTATIONS (Table 7.1)

Patients with nodules, vasculitis, neuropathy, Sjögren's syndrome and lung involvement are almost always rheumatoid factor positive.

Nodules

(*See* Table 7.2 for differential diagnosis of nodules in rheumatic diseases)
Firm subcutaneous lumps, ranging in size from barely palpable to several centimetres diameter. Often multiple. (Fig. 7.6)

Table 7.1　Non-articular manifestations of R A

System affected	Manifestation
General	Malaise, tiredness and depression (common)
	Anorexia and weight loss (less common)
	Fever (rare)
	Nodules (approx. 25%)
Vasomotor	Sweaty palms and skin atrophy
	Palmar erythema
	Raynaud's phenomenon (< 10%)
Haemopoietic	Anaemia
	Lymphadenopathy
	Splenomegaly
	Felty's syndrome
	Hyperviscosity syndrome
Vasculitis	Obliterative endarteritis
	Necrotising arteritis
	Leucocytoclastic vasculitis
Neurological	Entrapment neuropathy
	Peripheral neuropathy
	Mononeuritis multiplex
	Cervical myelopathy
Eye	Keratoconjunctivitis sicca
	Episcleritis and scleritis
	Scleromalacia perforans
Respiratory	Pleurisy and effusion
	Lung nodules
	Caplans syndrome
	Fibrosing alveolitis
Cardiac	Pericarditis
	Cardiac nodules
	Myocarditis

Table 7.2　Subcutaneous nodules in the rheumatic diseases

Rheumatoid arthritis	Characteristic nodule histology
Rheumatic fever ⎫	Nodule structure is less well organised and can
Still's disease ⎬	usually be distinguished from R A nodules
Gout	The 'nodule' is a tophus

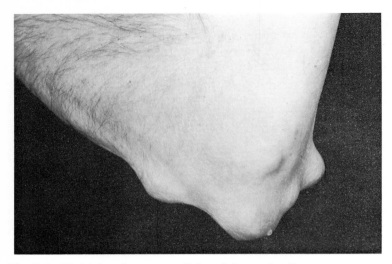

Fig. 7.6   Multiple subcutaneous RA nodules on the elbow.

Sites
Ulnar border of forearm near the elbow (most common).
In the walls of bursae especially the olecranon.
In tendons or their sheaths.
Any site of pressure: fingers, Achilles tendon, or sacrum.
Occasionally the eye or internal organs, e.g. heart or lung.

Haemopoietic

Anaemia (see p. 54). The commonest non-articular feature of RA and almost always accompanies active disease. It is of two types:
— anaemia of chronic disease: normochromic, normocytic
— iron deficiency anaemia.

Lymphadenopathy 30%. Usually associated with active synovitis. Glands are mobile, non-tender and rubbery. Histological picture of reactive hyperplasia.

Splenomegaly 5%.

Felty's syndrome 1% (Table 7.3). If associated with severe neutropenia, infection may be serious.

Hyperviscosity syndrome. A rare condition of increased serum viscosity, probably due to polymerization of macromolecules such as

Table 7.3 Features of Felty's syndrome

Features

Main:	Rheumatoid arthritis (seropositive)
	Splenomegaly
	Neutropenia
Other:	Lymphadenopathy
	Leg ulcers
	Pigmentation
	Weight loss
	Hepatomegaly
	Sjögren's syndrome
	Anaemia
	Thrombocytopenia

IgM, fibrinogen and rheumatoid factor and the formation of intermediate complexes of self-aggregating IgG RF. Causes dyspnoea, heart failure, epistaxis and impaired concentration and responds to plasmapheresis.

Drug-induced haemopoietic abnormalities. These include thrombocytopenia, leucopenia, and aplastic anaemia.

Vasculitis

Three major types are recognised:
1 Non-inflammatory obliterative endarteritis. This affects digital arteries causing small ischaemic lesions around the nail fold or in the finger pulp (Fig. 7.7), splinter haemorrhages, or rarely, digital gangrene.
2 Leucocytoclastic vasculitis may cause palpable purpura usually most prominent in the lower limbs.
3 Necrotising arteritis. A more serious lesion which may be histologically indistinguishable from polyarteritis nodosa. It is always associated with high titres of rheumatoid factor and usually with cryoproteins in the serum. It forms the pathological basis of the rare but serious syndrome known as malignant rheumatoid:
— purpura and skin ulceration
— gangrene of limbs or viscera especially gut
— peripheral neuropathy (motor type or mononeuritis multiplex)
— poor prognosis if not treated aggressively.

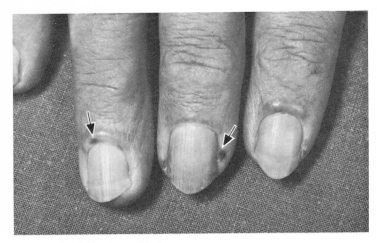

Fig. 7.7   Typical peiungal infarcts.

Neurological

Entrapment neuropathy:
— median nerve at the wrist is the most common type and may cause *carpal tunnel syndrome* (see below)
— ulnar nerves at the elbow
— posterior tibial nerve in the tarsal tunnel
— lateral popliteal nerve at the head of the fibula.
Peripheral neuropathy:
— sensory type.
Peripheral neuropathy:
— motor or mononeuritis multiplex type.
— caused by vasculitis.
Cervical myelopathy:
— This is caused by atlanto-axial subluxation
— or vertebral subluxation at a lower level, e.g. C3/4.

CARPAL TUNNEL SYNDROME

An entrapment neuropathy of the median nerve at the wrist which may be unilateral or bilateral is known as carpal tunnel syndrome.

Causes
— non-specific tenosynovitis
— rheumatoid arthritis

— pregnancy
— hypothyroidism
— amyloidosis
— acromegaly
— local trauma.

Symptoms (usually most marked at night)
— numbness and paraesthesiae in the lateral $3\frac{1}{2}$ fingers
— pain in the forearm, wrist or hand
— hand weakness.

Signs (often absent)
— weakness of thumb abduction and opposition
— wasting of thenar eminence
— sensory loss in median nerve distribution.

Diagnosis
— typical history
— nerve conduction studies may demonstrate prolonged conduction time across the wrist.

Treatment
— management of the cause
— immobilisation of the wrist by splinting
— local steroid injection
— surgical division of the transverse carpal ligament and flexor retinaculum to decompress median nerve.

Eye involvement

Keratoconjunctivitis sicca (*see* p. 167). This is the most common type of eye involvement and occurs in 10–30% of patients.
Episcleritis is a nodular or diffuse hyperaemia of the superficial sclera; it causes discomfort rather than pain and has a good prognosis.
Scleritis is an inflammation of the deeper layers of the sclera which is less common than episcleritis, but more serious. It heals with grey discolouration of the sclera.
Scleromalacia perforans is a rare but serious consequence of severe scleritis, scleral vasculitis, or nodule formation with sloughing of the affected area of sclera.
Iatrogenic drug-induced eye damage includes: steroid cataracts and chloroquine-induced corneal opacity or retinopathy.

Respiratory

Pleurisy and effusion. These are more common in males and often run a chronic course. The pleural fluid glucose is usually low.
Lung nodules are more common in males, usually peripheral, often just under the pleura, usually multiple and associated with nodules elsewhere, range in size from 0.5—3.0 cm in diameter, and may cavitate.
Caplan's syndrome is the association of rheumatoid nodules with pneumoconiosis; the nodules may be large and confluent.
Diffuse fibrosing alveolitis (Fig. 7.8) occurs more commonly in

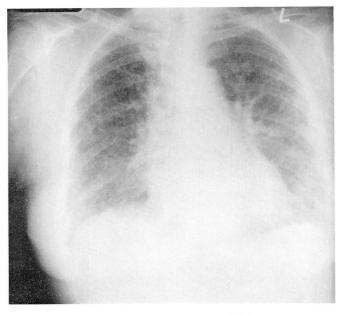

Fig. 7.8   Fibrosing alveolitis in rheumatoid arthritis.

RA than expected by chance but a causal relationship has not been established.
Obliterative bronchiolitis is a rare but serious, rapidly progressive obstructive disorder of the small airways.

Cardiac

Pericarditis is rarely of clinical importance, although echocardiography demonstrates small effusions in up to 50% of hospitalised patients with R A. Constrictive pericarditis is rare. Myocardial and endocardial nodules may result in conduction defects or valvular lesions.

COMPLICATIONS OF RHEUMATOID ARTHRITIS

Fracture of osteoporotic bones.

Septic arthritis. Damaged rheumatoid joints may act as a focus for infection, during bacteraemia. Symptoms and signs are often atypical and any rheumatoid patient who develops increased pain and swelling in one joint, with or without constitutional symptoms, should have the joint aspirated for culture without delay.

Amyloidosis. Often found at post mortem but of clinical significance in only a small number of patients. Is usually present as proteinuria and may be diagnosed by biopsy of kidney, rectal mucosa or fat.

Iatrogenic—drug-induced lesions include:
— eye: steroids, chloroquine
— blood: phenylbutazone, gold, penicillamine, immunosuppressives
— gastrointestinal: most anti-inflammatory drugs, steroids
— skin: most drugs
— kidney: gold, penicillamine
— liver: high dosage salicylates; other N S A I D.

8. Rheumatoid Arthritis: Laboratory Tests and Radiology

LABORATORY TESTS

Anaemia

Several causes are recognised:

Anaemia of chronic disease. This is the commonest cause of anaemia in RA. The degree of anaemia reflects disease activity and improves with control of disease. The range of haemoglobin in active disease is:

— males   10–14 g/dl
— females   9–12 g/dl.

Lower values than these suggest other causes.

Blood film: usually normochromic and normocytic, occasionally hypochromic and microcytic.

Serum iron: low; total iron binding capacity: low or normal.

Serum ferritin: normal or high.

Marrow iron stores: normal or increased.

Iron deficiency anaemia. This is commonly related to drug-induced gastrointestinal bleeding.

Serum iron studies are often unhelpful in diagnosis: serum iron is low and total iron binding capacity high but in the presence of active RA, the TIBC may be normal or low and results are therefore difficult to interpret.

Serum ferritin may not accurately reflect total body iron stores, since it acts as an acute phase reactant and may be elevated as a result of rheumatoid inflammation.

Confirmation of diagnosis requires demonstration of reduced iron stores by low serum ferritin or bone marrow examination.

Other causes include:

— folate deficiency (often dietary)
— haemolysis (very rare)
— sideroblastic anaemia (secondary to RA)
— marrow aplasia (drug induced).

Erythrocyte sedimentation rate

Generally elevated in RA and usually reflects the degree of disease activity. Elevation of the ESR disproportionate to disease activity may occur in:
— septic arthritis complicating RA
— longstanding, apparently 'burnt-out' disease
— intercurrent illnesses, e.g. myeloma, malignancy or infection
— amyloid.

White cell count (usually normal)

Leucocytosis may occur in:
— severe exacerbation of RA
— marked systemic disease, particularly vasculitis
— steroid treatment
— infection.
Leucopenia may occur in:
— drug-induced marrow depression
— Felty's syndrome (mainly neutropenia).

Platelet count (normal or elevated)

Thrombocytosis occurs in:
— active disease (may reach 1 million)
— acute bleeding.
Thrombocytopenia occurs in:
— drug-induced marrow depression
— Felty's syndrome.

Serum proteins

Alpha-2 and gammaglobulins often elevated.
Immunoglobulins, IgG, IgM and IgA may be individually or concurrently elevated.

Rheumatoid Factor (*see also* Chap. 5)

Positive in: 80% of patients by Latex test and 70% of patients by Rose Waaler test.
A positive test is *not* specific to RA, although it is uncommon to find very high titres in other conditions.

RF is usually associated with more severe disease and is almost invariably present in patients with nodules, Sjögren's syndrome, vasculitis, respiratory involvement and peripheral neuritis.

Antinuclear antibodies (*see also* Chap. 5)

Positive in 20–40% of patients, particularly those with Sjögren's syndrome.
No specific diagnostic or prognostic significance.

LE cells

Positive in 10% of patients.
Since this test detects just one of the ANA, the significance is the same as a positive ANA test.

Cryoproteins (*see* Chap. 5)

May be found in active vasculitis when the cryoproteins often contain rheumatoid factor.

Serum Complement (*see* Chap. 5)

Normal or elevated (in contrast to the *low synovial fluid* complement levels found in seropositive RA).

Synovial fluid (*see also* pp. 6–7)

Changes are non-specific and may be found in any inflammatory arthritis:
— volume: increased
— colour: yellow to opalescent
— clarity: translucent to opaque
— viscosity: low, due to reduced concentration of hyaluronate in inflammatory fluid
— protein: elevated (35–90 g/l)
— WCC: elevated (2000–100 000/cm^3), predominantly polymorphs, some contain immunoglobulin inclusions and are known as *ragocytes*
— glucose: reduced or normal
— rheumatoid factor: usually reflects serum but a positive test is not specific to RA
— complement: often reduced in seropositive RA.

Synovial biopsy

The histopathology of rheumatoid synovium is not pathognomonic.

Biopsy is rarely necessary in routine work-up except in monoarticular disease where other pathology, such as T B, requires exclusion.

Arthroscopy

Arthroscopy is a technique to visualise the joint interior using a fibreoptic arthroscope.

Rarely indicated in R A but is most useful in selecting a biopsy site in monoarticular disease.

RADIOLOGY

Changes vary with the stage of the disease.

In early disease:
— soft tissue swelling
— periarticular osteoporosis
— marginal erosions of bone (which initially occur at the junction of the synovium with the articular cartilage).

In later disease:
— progressive loss of joint space
— more extensive erosive changes and bone destruction
— joint subluxation or dislocation
— ankylosis (uncommon in R A except in the carpus)
— secondary degenerative changes.

Arthrography: contrast medium is injected into the joint and an X-ray taken. It is of value in the patient suspected of having a ruptured Baker's cyst and in the diagnosis of other synovial cysts.

Use of radiology

1 The routine investigation of a new patient should include X-rays of: hands and feet, chest; cervical spine, hips (pelvis) and knees if clinically involved.

2 The sites most likely to show early changes are: the feet and the hands and wrists.

3 Erosions provide the strongest support for a diagnosis of

RA; the absence of erosions in a patient with active synovitis of more than 3 years duration, raises suspicion of an alternate diagnosis.

4 Serial X-rays, at yearly intervals for example, provide a useful index of disease activity and response to treatment.

9. Rheumatoid Arthritis: Assessment, Management and Prognosis

ASSESSMENT

An accurate assessment of the patient with RA is an essential first step in devising a successful management plan. In the individual patient, the following questions must be answered:

1 Is the diagnosis correct?

The differential diagnosis of polyarthritis is also discussed in Chapter 4. The diagnosis of RA is a clinical one and there are no pathognomonic clinical or laboratory features.

Points favouring the diagnosis of RA:

— symmetrical polyarthritis
— prominent early morning stiffness
— nodules
— erosions on X-ray
— high titre rheumatoid factor.

Points against the diagnosis of RA:

— involvement of thoracic and lumbar spine
— skin, renal or CNS involvement
— negative RF with high titre ANA
— lack of erosions after several years active disease.

None of these necessarily excludes RA but may require explanation.

Monoarticular RA is well recognised but it should be investigated by examination of synovial fluid and tissue to exclude other causes, particularly infection.

2 What are the patient's problems and the pathology causing them?

The complaints of the rheumatoid patient may have several causes. The following are just three examples:

Pain may be due to:

— active synovitis
— secondary degenerative changes
— mechanical strain and ligamentous damage
— neuropathy.

Impaired hand function may be due to:
— active synovitis in the joints or flexor tendon sheaths
— inactive disease with joint subluxation, dislocation or fixed deformity
— ruptured tendons
— carpal tunnel syndrome
— marked wrist involvement.

Difficulty in walking may be due to:
— synovitis, erosion or subluxation of metatarsal heads
— muscle wasting and weakness
— fixed joint deformities
— peripheral neuropathy
— spasticity due to cervical myelopathy.

3   Is the disease active?
Pain alone is not necessarily a good guide to the presence of active synovitis since it may be just as severe in burnt-out disease.
Assessment of disease activity is critical since a major aim of drug therapy is the control of active synovitis. The best guides to the presence of active synovitis are:
— severity and duration of morning stiffness
— soft tissue swelling
— degree of 'anaemia of chronic disease'
— height of E S R
— prominent systemic symptoms including malaise, fatigue
— recent involvement of new joints
— radiological progression of erosions.

None of these points can be used in isolation as unequivocal evidence of active disease.

4   What is the degree of the patient's disability?
It is important to assess the effect of the disease on function:
— personal independence: toilet, bathing, dressing, eating, household tasks, shopping, cleaning
— mobility: around the house, stairs, public transport, car
— general activities and responsibilities: marriage, sexual activity, child care
— occupation.

MANAGEMENT

The main components of management are:
1 General measures: patient education, physical therapy, occupational therapy, appliances and footwear, social work.

2 Drug therapy.
3 Orthopaedic surgery.
4 Management of non-articular manifestations and special problems.

1 General measures

EDUCATION

For the majority of patients with RA, optimal treatment offers excellent prospects of disease control. The nature and wide spectrum of severity of the disease should be explained so that unjustified fears are allayed, the patient understands the purpose of the various steps in management, and has a realistic view of what can be achieved. Various publications, such as those available from arthritis organisations, provide patients with useful information which can form the basis for further discussion at later consultations. Education of the patient must be an ongoing process since only a limited amount of information is likely to be retained from a single consultation.

PHYSICAL THERAPY

Most patients require a physical therapy programme which is best planned and supervised by a physiotherapist.
Rest. Complete bed rest is necessary only for a minority of patients in the acute phase; unless correctly supervised, it may exacerbate muscle wasting and joint deformity. Splinting is used to rest joints and help prevent deformity:
— actively inflamed joints should be rested in a position of function, e.g. night wrist or knee splints
— painful, unstable wrists benefit from support in working splints
— serial splinting is used to correct early deformity, e.g. knee flexion.
Exercises. Correctly planned and graduated exercises are an essential part of management and are designed to preserve or improve the range of joint motion and to maintain or strengthen muscle power.
Types of exercise include:
— passive joint movement, which maintains the range of joint movement when actively inflamed joints are too painful for active exercises

— isometric exercises which preserve muscle power without stressing painful, inflamed joints

— active exercises against gravity or resistance to maintain range of joint movement and improve muscle power.

Other methods. Heat, cold, shortwave therapy, ultrasound, wax baths and hydrotherapy provide symptomatic relief of pain and stiffness, and allow the patient to undertake an exercise programme.

OCCUPATIONAL THERAPY

The occupational therapist is trained to assess and grade functional impairment and to devise methods to overcome the limitations imposed by disease and deformity.

The occupational therapist advises and assists in several areas:

— reduction of strain on involved joints

— adaptation of activities to improve function

— provision of aids and devices to assist the patient in personal and household tasks

— home visits to advise on simple adaptations and alterations.

For many patients with late disease and some disability, the occupational therapist is the person who provides most help.

APPLIANCES

Some of the more important items include:

— work splints for wrists, removable splints for unstable knees

— aids to mobility ranging from walking sticks to wheelchairs

— cervical collars ranging from soft collars for mild symptoms or use at night to firm collars for more severe symptoms or significant involvement, e.g. atlanto-axial subluxation

— special shoes and insoles are particularly useful since foot symptoms may be controlled without resort to drugs or surgery.

SOCIAL WORK

Social workers offer assistance with many of the domestic, financial, and occupational problems which confront the patient with a chronic, potentially disabling disease.

2 Drug therapy

Table 9.1   Drugs used in the treatment of rheumatoid arthritis

Analgesics:
  paracetamol
  dextropropoxyphene
  salicylates (low dose).
 	
Non-steroidal anti-inflammatory
drugs (NSAID):
  salicylate (high dose)
  indomethacin
  propionic acid derivatives
  many new agents.
 	
Anti-rheumatic drugs:
  gold
  D-penicillamine
  antimalarials
  sulphasalazine.
	Corticosteroids.
	
	Immunosuppressive drugs:
	  azathioprine
	  methotrexate
	  cyclophosphamide
	  chlorambucil.
	
	Intra-articular therapy:
	  corticosteroids
	  radioactive colloids.
	
	New and experimental therapy:
	  immunoregulatory drugs
	  new anti-rheumatic drugs.

Analgesics

Since analgesics relieve pain but have no anti-inflammatory effect their role in RA is limited.

Non-steroidal anti-inflammatory drugs (nsaid)

A wide and increasing range of these drugs is available. They fall within several chemical groups, some examples of which are shown in Table 9.2. They are the first line agents in the drug therapy of active synovitis since they combine analgesic and anti-inflammatory effects.

While they have not been shown to prevent erosions, they reduce pain and swelling and thereby allow better joint function. For many patients with mild disease they are sufficient to control symptoms and are the only drugs necessary.

Although the major members of the group have many similarities, it has been clearly shown that marked individual patient preferences occur. Thus failure to respond to one member of the group should not preclude therapeutic trial of other drugs in this category.

Table 9.2   Non-steroidal anti-inflammatory drugs

	Acidic agents		Non-acidic agents
Arylcarboxylic acids	Aryl alkanoic acids	Enolic acids	
Salicylic acids: acetylsalicylic acid (aspirin) diflunisal	Arylacetic acids: alclofenac diclofenac	Phenylbutazone Oxyphenbutazone Azapropazone	Proquazone Diftalone
Anthranilic acids (fenamates): flufenamic acid mefanamic acid meclofenamic acid	Arylpropionic acids: ibuprofen naproxen ketoprofen fenoprofen		
	Heteroarylacetic acids: tolmetin fenclozic acid		
	Indole and indene acetic acids: indomethacin sulindac		

MODE OF ACTION

Prostaglandin synthetase inhibition is one effect which is considered important in the suppression of inflammation and is common to many drugs in this group. Other mechanisms are probably involved. Aspirin, for example, has a central antipyretic action and both central and peripheral analgesic effects. It may also affect lymphokine production or action, neutrophil adhesion to vascular endothelium, fibrinolysis, the activation of kallikrein and the localisation of immune complexes through its inhibition of platelet aggregation.

INDICATIONS FOR USE

The indications are active synovitis and pain due to secondary degenerative changes which does not respond to simple analgesics.

SALICYLATES

Clinical use   There are four main points:
1   To produce an optimal anti-inflammatory effect, the serum salicylate level should be maintained within the therapeutic range (15–30 mg%; 1–2 mmol/l).
2   Adults usually require 4 g or more daily; the frequency of administration depends on the formulation. Measurement of serum salicylate levels is the most reliable method by which to adjust the dose.
3   Patients show considerable variability in the salicylate level produced by standard doses of any one preparation and if one formulation fails to achieve therapeutic blood levels, another may prove effective.
4   If side effects develop at blood levels below the therapeutic range, it is better to change to an alternate N S A I D.
Note:
Salicylates are now being replaced by newer non-steroidal agents.

Side effects and drug interactions   Side effects of salicylates are shown in Table 9.3 and important drug interactions are shown in Table 9.4.
Dyspepsia is the commonest side effect of salicylate therapy, reported to occur in up to 30% of patients.
Gastric erosions and bleeding are common but do not correlate with dyspeptic symptoms.
Gastrointestinal side effects are minimised by using aloxoprin, slow release or enteric coated preparations.
Tinnitus and deafness are common early symptoms of toxicity but may occur when salicylate levels are well within the therapeutic range, particularly in older patients.
Perhaps the greatest problem with salicylates is their lack of popularity. Their familiarity as well as the high frequency of gastric disturbances cause low patient compliance.

PROPIONIC ACID DERIVATIVES

Clinical use   Many rheumatologists now use one of these drugs, in preference to aspirin, as the first choice within the N S A I D group since they are effective, well tolerated, and have a low incidence of side effects.
Since patients show variability in their response to these agents,

Table 9.3   Salicylate side effects.

Gastrointestinal upset
dyspepsia, nausea and vomiting
gastric erosions and blood loss
peptic ulceration

Tinnitus and deafness
may occur at salicylate levels over 1.3 mmol/l or at lower levels in older patients

Bruising and bleeding
inhibition of platelet aggregation
hypoprothrombinaemia (rarely)

Hypersensitivity reaction
especially in patients with nasal polyps and asthma
severe asthma
urticaria
anaphylactic shock

Salicylism (overdose)
tinnitus and deafness
stimulation of respiration leading to hyperventilation and respiratory alkalosis
other signs include nausea, vomiting, vertigo, flushing, sweating, and tachycardia
respiratory and cardiovascular depression leading to respiratory and metabolic acidosis with attendant fever, confusion, convulsions, coma and respiratory failure

---

Table 9.4   Salicylate drug interactions

Other drugs	Interaction
Oral anticoagulants Oral hypoglycaemics	Potentiated
Antacids Steroids	Reduce salicylate levels
Uricosurics	Inhibited by low dose salicylates
Alcohol	Increased gastric irritation

it is often necessary to undertake a therapeutic trial of successive members of the group to find the drug which best suits the individual patient.
There is rarely any advantage in using more than one of these drugs simultaneously.
These drugs potentiate oral anticoagulants.

Preparations and administration (Table 9.5).

Table 9.5 Propionic acid derivatives (some examples)

Drug	Formulation		Administration
Ibuprofen	Tablets	200 mg	400 mg tds or qds
		400 mg	
Naproxen	Tablets	250 mg	250–500 mg bd
Fenoprofen	Tablets or		300–600 mg qds
	capsules	300 mg	
Ketoprofen*	Capsules	50 mg	50 mg tds
	Suppositories	100 mg	100 mg nocte

* A slow-release preparation is now available

Side effects These include gastrointestinal effects (dyspepsia and nausea or occasional gastrointestinal bleeding), hypersensitivity reactions (exacerbation of asthma has been reported in some patients with aspirin hypersensitivity).

INDOMETHACIN

Clinical use An effective anti-inflammatory analgesic which is particularly useful for the relief of morning stiffness. Its use is limited by the high incidence of gastrointestinal and central nervous system side effects which occur in up to 30% of patients, particularly the elderly.

Preparations and administration Capsules 25 mg, slow release 75 mg capsules, suppositories 100 mg.
Dose: 25 mg 2–4 times daily with food, 50–100 mg at night taken orally or as a suppository.
A slow release preparation, 75 mg once or twice daily, has been introduced and is proving a well tolerated drug.
To minimise side effects, it is advisable to introduce indomethacin at low dosage, initially at night, and gradually to increase the dose over 1–2 weeks; capsules should be taken with food.

Side effects   These are of four main varieties:
Gastrointestinal (common)
— dyspepsia, abdominal pain, anorexia and nausea
— gastric erosions and bleeding
— peptic ulceration common when used with steroids. (Ulcers occur particularly in the prepyloric region and sometimes resemble malignant ulcers on barium meal).
Central nervous system (common)
— headaches, vertigo and dizziness
— heavy 'foggy' heads
— depression
— nightmares.
Hypersensitivity reactions (rare)
— may occur in patients with aspirin hypersensitivity.
Fluid retention, exacerbation of hypertension and antagonism to diuretics and anti-hypertensives.

SULINDAC

Clinical use   An indene derivative with analgesic and anti-inflammatory effects, a low incidence of side effects and a long half-life allowing twice daily administration. There is evidence that in contrast to most N S A I D, sulindac does not inhibit renal prostaglandins and in patients with mild renal impairment, it does not reduce glomerular filtration or renal plasma flow.

Preparation and administration
Tablets 100 mg
Dose: 100–200 mg bd.

Side effects   These are gastrointestinal and occur in up to 25% of patients. They include dyspepsia, nausea, and constipation. Hepatoxicity is reported.

PHENYLBUTAZONE AND OXYPHENBUTAZONE

Clinical use   These two drugs are sufficiently similar to be regarded as the same substance with respect to their therapeutic use and side effects. They are powerful analgesic, anti-inflammatory drugs but their rare, potentially serious side effects should limit their use to special situations.

They should not be used in combination with gold, D-penicillamine or other drugs which may also cause marrow depression.

Preparations and administration
Phenylbutazone tablets 100 to 200 mg, suppositories 250 mg, i.m. injection 600 mg/3 ml.
Dose: tablets 100–400 mg daily taken with food.
Side effects   Side effects occur in 20–30% of patients and drug interactions are particularly important. They include gastrointestinal effects such as nausea, vomiting and dyspepsia, peptic ulceration and bleeding, or diarrhoea; skin rashes and hypersensitivity reactions; haematological effects such as aplastic anaemia (most commonly in older patients on long-term therapy), and neutropenia, thrombycytopenia and agranulocytosis (more common in younger patients and usually within 3 months of starting treatment); salt and water retention which may precipitate cardiac failure in susceptible patients and antagonise diuretic and antihypertensive therapy; and drug interactions including marked potentiation of oral anticoagulants and oral hypoglycaemics.

OTHER NON-STEROIDALS

It is appropriate to select only a few examples of N S A I D for further comment.

Fenamates (flufenamic acid and mefanamic acid) are analgesics with slight anti-inflammatory effects.
Dosage: flufenamic acid: 100–200 mg tds, meranamic acid: 250–500 mg tds
Side effects include: gastrointestinal disturbances, (especially diarrhoea), exacerbation of asthma in aspirin-sensitive patients, and potentiation of oral anticoagulants.

Arylacetic acids (alclofenac, dicofenac and fenclofenac) are analgesics with anti-inflammatory effects; it has been claimed, but not established, that alclofenac and fenclofenac may have a suppressive effect on the activity of rheumatoid synovitis.
Dosage: diclofenac: 25–50 mg bd or tds, fenclofenac: 300 mg bd-qds
Side effects include: gastrointestinal disturbances, skin rashes, potentiation of oral anticoagulants and hypoglycaemics.

Anti-rheumatic drugs

These include gold (sodium aurothiomalate, aurothioglucose), D-penicillamine, chloroquine, and hydroxychloroquine.

GENERAL PROPERTIES

They are non-analgesic.

Onset of action is slow: usually 10–20 weeks of treatment are necessary before full effectiveness becomes evident.

They are significantly more toxic than the NSAID: their administration requires close supervision and monitoring with appropriate laboratory tests.

Up to 70% of patients show improvement, to a variable degree, in synovitis, some non-articular features and laboratory measurements such as Hb and ESR.

These drugs suppress rheumatoid disease activity and there is evidence that they prevent or slow the rate of erosive changes and improve the prognosis.

They do not cure rheumatoid arthritis; continued suppression of disease activity requires continued administration.

Their precise mode of action is unclear.

Indications Active rheumatoid arthritis not responding to optimal therapy with non-steroidal anti-inflammatory drugs.

Note:

Opinions differ on the timing of introduction of these agents but, once the diagnosis is established, they should be given before irreversiable joint damage has occurred.

Which drug to use? At present, the choice usually lies between gold and D-penicillamine. There is no clear evidence favouring one over the other in terms of efficacy. Gold has the advantage of long experience of use but requires regular injections. Antimalarials, although used in SLE, are less widely used in rheumatoid arthritis.

GOLD (Sodium aurothiomalate, sodium aurothioglucose).

Gold has been used in the management of RA since 1927. It remains one of the most valuable drugs available for the control of rheumatoid arthritis and, although associated with a formidable list of potential toxic effects, serious problems are minimised by carefully supervised and monitored administration. Its mechanism of action in RA is still unclear although it has powerful effects on macrophages and may prevent the release of lysosomal enzymes.

Administration and dosage Gold is given by intramuscular injection. Administration regimens vary:

Test dose: 5–10 mg i.m.
Weekly dose: 20–50 mg i.m. to a total dose of 0.5–1.0 g
Maintenance therapy: 10–50 mg i.m. every 2–4 weeks.
When using this scheme it should be noted that:
Assessment of response is based on clinical criteria.
Serum gold levels provide little help in assessing the likely response and no help in predicting toxic effects.
If the patient shows improvement, maintenance therapy is continued long term.
If the patient has not responded after receiving 1.0 g of gold, the drug is usually stopped.
If toxic effects develop, gold is stopped although it is often possible, cautiously, to re-introduce it.
Gold should not be given with other drugs which may also cause bone marrow depression, e.g. phenylbutazone or immunosuppressives.

Clinical and laboratory monitoring of administration.
The patient must be aware of potential side effects and report any adverse reactions immediately.
Before each injection, the patient must be asked about pruritus, skin rashes and mouth ulcers.
Urinalysis for proteinuria should be performed before each injection.
Full blood count, including a platelet count must be performed regularly, ideally before each gold injection or at least monthly.
It is advisable to keep a gold progress chart which serially records the gold dose, progressive total gold dose, and the results of the urinalysis, Hb, W C C, platelet count and E S R.

Side effects   These occur in up to 30% of patients. They are of four main types:
1   Mucocutaneous (most common)
Rash
— almost invariably preceded and accompanied by pruritus
— usually occurs within the first few months of treatment (often around a total dose of 300 mg)
— form and site of rash are variable; any pruritic rash developing during treatment must be attributed, at least provisionally, to gold
— continued administration of gold may produce an exfoliative dermatitis

— resolves on gold withdrawal; sometimes within weeks, sometimes slowly over months.

Mouth ulcers
— may accompany skin rash or occur alone
— often indistinguishable from aphthous ulcers.

2 Nephropathy
Proteinuria
— may occur transiently in 10% of patients.

Nephrotic syndrome
— renal lesion is a membranous nephritis
— resolves slowly on gold withdrawal.

3 Haematological (rare but serious) and include:
Thrombocytopenia
— may occur suddenly after one or two injections
— may be reversible but fatalities have occurred.

Leukopenia and marrow aplasia
— occurs more slowly, usually after a progressive fall in the WCC (stressing the importance of a WCC card or record)
— poor prognosis.

Eosinophilia
— may occur with or without skin rash.

4 Other side effects (uncommon)
— transient vasomotor reactions following injections
— post-injection arthralgia
— diarrhoea, due to enterocolitis
— 'gold lung', i.e., gold induced pulmonary infiltration.

ORAL GOLD

An oral preparation of a gold salt Auranofin is currently undergoing worldwide trials. Despite occasional troublesome diarrhoea, the therapeutic results look promising.

D-PENICILLAMINE

This is a degradation product of penicillin. Its effect on rheumatoid arthritis and its side effects are similar to those of gold; administration requires the same precautions.

Although originally introduced because penicillamine is capable of dissociating sulphydryl bonds and reducing the titre of rheumatoid factor, it is now recognised that this is not the mechanism by which it exerts its effect on rheumatoid arthritis.

D-penicillamine appears to have both chemical and immunological effects but its precise mode of action is unknown.

Administration and dosage
Formulation: tablets 125 and 250 mg
Dose: side effects are reduced by introducing D-penicillamine at
low dose, increasing the dose gradually, and using a relatively low
maintenance dose.
Initial dose: 125–250 mg daily
Increase dose by 125–250 mg every 4–8 weeks
Maintenance dose: 500–750 mg daily

It should be noted that:
The maintenance dose is that at which the patient shows improvement.
If a response has not occurred on 750–1000 mg daily, the drug is
usually stopped.
Mild side effects may be relieved by reducing the dose and subsequently increasing it more slowly.
Blood levels of penicillamine are not yet generally available and
their assistance in guiding therapy is uncertain at present.

Side effects   These occur in up to 50% of patients but require
cessation of therapy less frequently than those caused by gold.
They are of six main types:
1   Gastrointestinal side effects are uncommon if the drug is
introduced as low dose and increased slowly
— anorexia and nausea (these occur early)
— taste loss or alteration.
2   Mucucutaneous (common)
Rash
— may be either early (within first 6 months of treatment, maculopapular, transient, and does not usually recur with re-
   introduction of treatment) or late (occurs, usually, after more
   than 6 months of treatment, less common than early rash,
   pruritic, scaly plaques, settles slowly on withdrawal, and
   usually recurs on re-introduction of drug)
Mouth ulcers
— occur in about 5% of patients; may be severe and require
   permanent withdrawal of drug.
3   Nephropathy
Proteinuria
— common (about 15%), occurs after about 4 months of treat-

ment, and although progression to nephrotic syndrome is rare, persistent proteinurea (3–4 weeks) suggests withdrawal of the drug

Nephrotic syndrome
— the renal lesion is an immune complex membranous nephritis and gradually resolves on withdrawal of the drug.

4   Haematological disorders

Thrombocytopenia
— common (about 15%), less serious than gold-induced thrombocytopenia since it recovers rapidly on withdrawal.

Neutropenia and marrow aplasia
— rare but serious.

5   Febrile reactions (rare).

6   Other side effects (rare and usually occur late)
— drug induced lupus erythematosus
— myasthenia gravis and polymyositis
— Goodpasture's syndrome
— pemphigus.

CHLOROQUINE AND HYDROXYCHLOROQUINE

The antimalarials have a delayed suppressive effect on rheumatoid arthritis like gold and penicillamine, but are less effective. Retinopathy is a potential side effect of the antimalarials, particularly chloroquine, although this rarely develops if the patient has normal renal function and takes the recommended dose. Concerns about this complication have limited the long-term use of these drugs in RA.

Administration and dosage

Formulations:
Chloroquine phosphate 250 mg tablets
Chloroquine sulphate 200 mg tablets
Hydroxychloroquine sulphate 200 mg tablets

Dose:
Chloroquine 4 mg/kg/day to a maximum dose of 250 mg daily
Hydroxychloroquine 6 mg/kg/day to a maximum dose of 400 mg daily.

It should be noted that:
Ophthalmological examination, including visual fields for red scotoma, must be carried out before treatment is commenced and at six-monthly intervals during treatment.

Patients should be warned to report any visual symptoms. In patients with a reduced creatinine clearance, the daily dose should be reduced and long-term therapy is probably inadvisable. Antimalarials are contraindicated in pregnancy.

Side effects   These are of three main types:
1   Ocular
Retinopathy
— dose related, irreversible, initially detected by development of a red scotoma and corneal opacities which are reversible.
2   Skin rash
— including depigmentation and alopecia
3   Myopathy

Corticosteroids

Steroids stand in a category of their own as the most potent anti-inflammatory agents available. There is, however, little evidence that they have beneficial long-term effects on the course of the disease. Their suppressive effect on rheumatoid disease is dramatic but they are difficult to withdraw without disease exacerbation. Since rheumatoid arthritis is a chronic illness, introduction of steroids may commit the patient to long term therapy, which, even in modest doses, may cause many side effects.

Despite these difficulties, steroids have a place in the management of RA and it is possible to use them effectively and safely.

INDICATIONS AND USE

Costeroid therapy is clearly indicated when life or individual organs are threatened by steroid-responsive disease, e.g. vasculitis or pericarditis. Steroids should be given in sufficient dose to suppress disease activity, i.e. 60–80 mg per day.

The relative indications include the patient with very active disease, despite a full non-steroidal anti-inflammatory drug regimen, who has been commenced on an anti-rheumatic drug. Low dose steroids provide some relief during the interval before gold or penicillamine becomes effective. When the anti-rheumatic drug begins to bring the disease under control, steroid can be reduced at a rate of about 1 mg per month. Also for the very elderly patient, already incapacitated by the infirmity of age, who develops acute rheumatoid arthritis and suffers severe functional impairment, or the patient who fails to respond to an anti-rheumatic drug, a small dose of steroid may be used before or with an immunosuppressive.

If steroids are used in these situations the following guidelines should generally be observed:

— use the smallest dose able to produce a beneficial rather than totally suppressive effect, e.g. 5–10 mg daily
— single morning dose preferable
— the therapeutic plan should allow slow but persistent reduction in dose, aiming at ultimate withdrawal.

SIDE EFFECTS

The major side effects are listed in Table 9.6.

Table 9.6   Side effects of corticosteroids

System affected	Side effect
Endocrine	Cushingoid features:moon face, truncal obesity, buffalo hump, hirsuitism
	Hyperglycaemia; diabetes
	Adrenal insufficiency
Skin	Facial erythema
	Thinning and bruising
	Striae
Musculoskeletal	Myopathy
	Osteoporosis
	Aseptic necrosis
Gastrointestinal	Peptic ulceration
Eye	Posterior subcapsular cataracts
Central nervous system	Alterations in mood
	Psychoses
	Benign intracranial hypertension
Immunological	Immune suppression
	Increased susceptibility to infection
Cardiovascular system	Fluid retention
	Hypertension

Immunosuppressives

These drugs, although very effective in rheumatoid arthritis, are not suitable for general use and cannot be regarded as a routine form of management. The high incidence of side effects and the potential dangers of long-term immunosuppression demand very careful consideration before they are used to treat this non-fatal condition. Their use should be limited to specialist units familiar with their administration, monitoring and toxic effects.

INDICATIONS

Severe, progressive disease which is not controlled by the anti-rheumatic drugs either because they are ineffectual or produce side effects which prevent their further use.
Note:
This relative indication must balance the dangers of immunosup-pressives against a variety of factors including the patient's age, sex, disease progression and function.

SIDE EFFECTS

Marrow depression (dose related leukopenia most common).
Increased susceptibility to infection (particularly herpes zoster and infection with unusual organisms and fungi).
Gastrointestinal effects (anorexia, nausea, vomiting).
Increased incidence of malignancy (especially haematological).
Chromosomal and mutagenic effects (?).

Particular side effects of individual drugs include occasional hepatotoxicity (azathioprine), haemorrhagic cystitis, bladder fi-brosis, alopecia (cyclophosphamide), stomatitis and infertility (cyclophosphamide and chlorambucil).

AZATHIOPRINE

This is an antimetabolite which interferes with purine biosyn-thesis.
It is effective in up to 80% of patients with RA.
Onset of action slow.
It is also considerably less toxic than cyclophosphamide and therefore easier to use.

CYCLOPHOSPHAMIDE

This is an alkylating agent with a more rapid onset of action than azathioprine.
It is highly effective in treating rheumatoid arthritis but asso-ciated with side effects in about 90% of patients.
Its use is reserved for special, severe situations.

CHLORAMBUCIL

This alkylating agent, similar to cyclophosphamide, has fewer short-term side effects. As with cyclophosphamide, leukaemia and other malignancies may be late complications.

Intra-articular therapy

CORTICOSTEROIDS

Locally administered corticosteroids provide anti-inflammatory activity but avoid the side effects of systemic steroids. They are therefore most appropriately used for *localised* problems, resulting from inflammation which has not been otherwise controlled.

The benefits of local steroids are unpredictable: some patients show transient improvement while others have a more lasting response. If the initial injection is unsuccessful a second is warranted; if this fails, the problem requires a different approach. Although the dangers of local steroids have probably been over-emphasised, multiple injections into the same joint are unjustifiable.

Indications
Intra-articular:
— for pain or swelling due to inflammation
— for remobilisation of a stiff joint.
Into tendon sheaths:
— for tenosynovitis, especially of the finger flexors.
Into soft tissues:
— carpal tunnel for entrapment neuropathy
— bursae.
Note:
Intra-articular steroids must never be given if there is any possibility of joint infection and injections must always be carried out under aseptic conditions.

RADIOACTIVE COLLOIDS

Radioactive synovectomy, performed by the intra-articular injection of a radioactive isotope, such as ^{90}Yttrium has been used for the control of localised synovitis which has failed to respond to systemic measures.

New and experimental therapy

Several other drugs have been shown to exert to a variable extent a suppressive effect on R A synovitis. These include levamisole, sulphasalazine and dapsone; their role as routine therapeutic agents awaits further evaluation. A variety of methods have been used to manipulate the immune system. These include lymphocyte depletion by thoracic duct drainage and lymphopheresis, removal of putative immune complexes by plasmapheresis, and total lymphoid irradiation. At present, these approaches are experimental but some may point the way to further advances.

3 Orthopaedic surgery

Surgery is of value in the management of local structural problems involving joints or soft tissues when these have failed to respond to medical measures. Decisions regarding surgery in R A are often difficult and combined rheumatology/orthopaedic clinics are important. Some of the more important operations in R A are:
1 Removal of metatarsal heads (Fowler's or Hoffman's operations). A most successful procedure for painful eroded subluxed M T P joints.
2 Total hip replacement. A very successful operation for severe hip involvement; best results are obtained when other lower limb joints are minimally affected.
3 Total knee replacement. Although somewhat less satisfactory than total hip replacement, the newer total knee prostheses have an acceptable success rate.
4 Hand and wrist surgery. Flexor tendon clearance, ulnar styloidectomy and stabilisation of the wrist and some small joints of the hand usefully improve function. Synovectomy and finger joint replacements require careful patient selection since their long term success is variable.
5 Cervical spine. Fusion is indicated in patients with instability causing cord compression or severe pain which is uncontrolled by other measures.
6 Synovectomy of the knee. This procedure is becoming less popular; short term relief of pain and effusion is outweighed by the long term development of secondary degenerative changes and recurrence of inflammatory synovitis.
7 Synovectomy of elbow and excision of the radial head is a

useful procedure for the relief of pain in advanced disease of the elbow.

4   Management of non-articular manifestations and special problems

ANAEMIA

The anaemia of chronic disease generally responds only to adequate control of the rheumatoid disease. Haematinic agents are unhelpful. Superimposed iron deficiency anaemia is also common in RA. Management involves investigation and treating the cause (usually GI blood loss); together with iron supplements.

NODULES

These are rarely painful and generally require no treatment. These may regress with local steroid injection or control of disease. Excision is sometimes followed by recurrence of the nodule.

SICCA SYNDROME (*see* Chapter 15)

ACTIVE DISEASE IN THE PATIENT WITH A PEPTIC ULCER

There are no entirely safe solutions to this problem. The early use of an antirheumatic drug is indicated but the problem period is the interval before the gold or D-penicillamine becomes effective.

In the presence of an active peptic ulcer, none of the NSAID can be endorsed as safe drugs. The use of an H2 antagonist, cimetidine or ranitidine, is often required.

Further management of symptoms and synovitis may include a simple analgesic e.g. paracetamol for mild pain and prednisone 5–10 mg daily without *any* other anti-inflammatory drugs for very active disease. Perhaps surprisingly, prednisolone has less ulcer-causing potential than most of the NSAID's.

COURSE AND PROGNOSIS

For the patient with early RA, there are no accurate guides as to the course the disease will follow. Although there is marked individual variation, the following features are associated with a worse prognosis:
— insidious onset
— persistent disease activity

— young age at onset
— seropositivity
— early erosive changes
— marked systemic features.

DISEASE ACTIVITY PATTERNS

Two main patterns of disease activity are recognised: *persistent* (75-80% of patients) and *intermittent* or *episodic* activity (20-25% of patients). In the second type, episodes of arthritis generally last 6-12 months and remissions may last months or years. Some patients progress to persistent disease. An episode of arthritis lasting for more than 3 years rarely goes into complete remission.

Monoarticular disease progresses to polyarticular arthritis in about 40% of patients within ten years.

PROGNOSIS

Most reported figures on prognosis are biased towards hospital populations; many patients with mild RA are never seen in outpatient departments and their prognosis appears to be good. In terms of function, a rough guide to the ultimate outcome is:
— 50% have little disability
— 40% show moderate to severe disability
— 10% become severely disabled.
Death due to rheumatoid arthritis is uncommon but does occur. The major causes are: progressive systemic disease, infection, or amyloidosis.

10 Seronegative Arthropathies

The term *seronegative arthropathies*, or *seronegative spondarthritides*, conventionally includes the following entities:
Ankylosing spondylitis
Reiter's syndrome
Psoriatic arthritis and spondylitis
Enteropathic arthritis and spondylitis
Juvenile chronic arthritis (*see* Chap. 11).
These disorders; although clinically distinct and usually easily separated, are unified by two major characteristics: the synovial histology of involved peripheral joints may be indistinguishable from RA but rheumatoid factor is absent.

In addition, there are several features which occur commonly in each entity within the group: sacroiliitis and spondylitis, iritis, mucocutaneous lesions, familial aggregation of single and occasionally multiple seronegative arthropathies, and increased prevalence of HLA-B27. Thus the several clinical features shared by this group of rheumatic diseases appear to be linked by a common genetic thread.

ANKYLOSING SPONDYLITIS

Ankylosing spondylitis (AS) is a chronic inflammatory arthritis which principally affects the axial skeleton but also commonly involves the peripheral joints, particularly the shoulders and lower limb joints. Spinal movement becomes restricted and in advanced disease, apophyseal joint fusion, syndesmophyte formation and calcification of spinal ligaments may cause complete rigidity from the neck to the sacrum. A pathological and clinical condition similar or identical to AS may occur with Reiter's syndrome, psoriasis and psoriatic arthritis or inflammatory bowel disease.

Epidemiology

Prevalence Varies in different races. Estimated to affect 0.5–2.0% of Caucasian males; a lower figure is probably correct. Incomplete forms of the disease may be more common.

Sex Male:female: ratio 5:1; some recent surveys suggest ratio is nearer 2:1.

Age Onset usually second and third decades.

Family history Up to 7% of the first degree relatives of probands also have ankylosing spondylitis, i.e. their risk is increased about twenty times. Some families show an increased prevalence of inflammatory bowel disease, psoriasis and Reiter's syndrome.

Aetiology

The cause of A S is unknown but genetic and environmental factors appear important.

GENETIC FACTORS

Familial aggregation of A S and other seronegative arthropathies. H L A-B27 association: B27 is present in >90% of patients with A S. When A S occurs with psoriasis or inflammatory bowel disease, H L A-B27 is present in only about 60% of patients. This suggests that the genes which contribute to these disorders reduce the need for H L A-B27 in the development of A S.

ENVIRONMENTAL FACTORS

Identical twins who are discordant for the disease indicate a contribution from environmental factors. An infectious agent is suspected but not proven to play some role in pathogenesis.

Pathology

There appear to be two basic pathological processes operating in A S:

1 Synovitis—which may be identical histologically to that in R A.

2 Enthesopathy—this term refers to an inflammatory reaction at the *enthesis* which is the zone of ligamentous attachment to bone.

The synovitis shows a more prominent progression to ankylosis than is seen in RA and the enthesopathy, particularly in the spine, progresses to ligamentous ossification.

SITES AFFECTED

Axial joints. (sacroiliac, spinal apophyseal and costovertebral). These joints show a combination of synovitis and enthesopathy which progresses to bony ankylosis of the joint periphery and later to central endochondral ossification.

Intervertebral discs. The major process around the disc is an enthesopathy with inflammatory changes occurring initially at the insertion of the annulus fibrosus at the vertebral margin. This progresses to calcification of the outer layer of the annulus thereby producing the bony bridge between the vertebral bodies, known as a 'syndesmophyte' (Fig. 10.1). The earliest syndesmophytes usually occur at the thoracolumbar junction. When they develop extensively along the spine, they cause bony rigidity and the typical 'bamboo' appearance on X-ray. The latter is accentuated by calcification of the longitudinal spinal ligaments which occurs later in established disease. Involvement of the symphysis

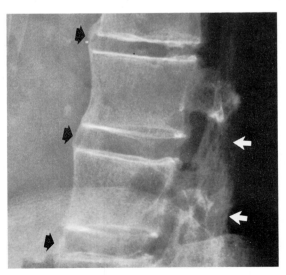

Fig. 10.1 Lateral view of the lumbar spine syndesmophyte formation (black arrows). There is bony alkylosis of the apophyseal joints (white arrows) completing the fusion. (Dr David Lewall, King Faisal Specialist Hospital, Saudi Arabia.)

pubis and the manubriosternal joints, both of which are cartilaginous, is probably similar to the process at the intervertebral disc.

Peripheral Joints. Synovitis is nonspecific and may be identical to that seen in RA except that it tends more readily to progress to bony ankylosis.

Tendinous insertions. Enthesopathy frequently occurs at the sites of ligamentous attachments particularly around ischial tuberosities, the greater and lesser trochanters of the femur and the iliac crests. When calcification occurs at these sites it causes a characteristic 'whiskering' appearance on X-ray. Other sites which can be similarly affected include:

— insertion of the plantar fascia
— Achilles tendon at the heel
— insertion of the patella ligament into the tibial tuberosity.

Clinical features

ONSET

Onset is usually insidious. Low back pain and stiffness are the most common presentation. Peripheral arthritis, usually of the lower limb, is the presenting feature in 15–20% of cases. The younger the age of onset the more likely a peripheral joint presentation, particularly of the hip, knee or ankle. Systemic malaise, tiredness, anorexia and weight loss may accompany active disease but are rarely as prominent as in RA.

ARTICULAR MANIFESTATIONS

Low back.
Pain and stiffness are usually most marked in the low back but may occur predominantly in the thoracolumbar region. Early morning stiffness in the low back and buttocks is prominent, often severe and prolonged.
Pain:
— often radiates to buttocks or posterior thighs but rarely below the knees
— unaccompanied by paraesthesiae or neurological signs
— may move from side to side
— unrelieved by rest
— often most troublesome at night and in the early hours of the

morning, waking the patient from sleep and forcing him to walk around to relieve aching stiffness
— relieved by moderate activity but strenuous back strain usually causes exacerbation
— commonly epidosic, lasting days or weeks and then improving spontaneously for a period.

Symptoms of inflammatory spondylitis are usually easily distinguished from mechanical back lesions which are characterised by pain which is:
— relieved by rest
— worsened by bending and lifting
— accompanied by stiffness which may be severe but is transient
— sometimes accompanied by paraesthesiae and neurological signs of nerve root irritation.

Early signs may include:
— loss of normal lumbar lordosis due to muscle spasm
— sacroiliac joint tenderness
— restriction of movement in all three planes, i.e. flexion, extension and lateral flexion.

Later signs include:
— kyphosis
— marked limitation or complete rigidity of spine
— absence of sacroiliac joint tenderness.

Cervical and thoracic spine
Pain and stiffness occur in the neck and thoracic area.
Typical complaints include:
— pain between the shoulder blades
— pain around the chest especially on sneezing and coughing due to costovertebral joint involvement.

Signs include:
— loss of movement in the cervical spine
— restriction of chest expansion (to <5 cm at the level of the fourth intercostal space).

OTHER ARTICULAR FEATURES

Other central joints which may be affected include sternoclavicular, manubriosternal and symphysis pubis joints.
Peripheral joint involvement:
— occurs in 50% of patients at some time during the course of the disease

— affects particularly the shoulders, hips, knees, ankles and small joints of feet.
— it is often asymmetrical.
— in the absence of Reiter's syndrome or psoriasis, involvement of the wrists and small joints of the hands is rare
— often severe and erosive with a tendency to ankylosis, producing severe disability especially at the hips and shoulders.

Enthesopathy at the sites of tendon insertions and muscle attachments frequently involve:
— plantar surface of heels — *plantar fasciitis*
— attachment of the thigh adductors at the pelvis
— the ischial tuberosity
— the pelvic brim.

NON-ARTICULAR MANIFESTATIONS

Iritis may occur in up to 25% of patients. It is unrelated to the severity or activity of spondylitis.

Cardiac involvement is uncommon, occurring in 2–8% of patients and causing conduction defects, aortic incompetence or pericarditis.

Apical pulmonary fibrosis, resembling T B, is well recognised but rare.

Neurological involvement such as a cauda equina lesion, probably due to chronic arachnoiditis, is very rare.

Other Diseases. Since ankylosing spondylitis may occur in the other seronegative arthropathies, the patient presenting with what appears to be typical A S may be found to have evidence of psoriasis, inflammatory bowel disease, or Reiter's syndrome.

COMPLICATIONS

Spinal fractures: when the spine is rigid, trauma more easily causes fractures which are always serious and may be fatal.
Amyloidosis is rare

Laboratory tests

Haematology
Hb: normochromic, normocytic anaemia may occur but in contrast to R A, patients with active disease often have a normal haemoglobin and blood film.

E S R: elevated in active disease in about 70% of patients but does not correlate well with variations in activity of the spondylitis.

HLA-B27
Present in >90% of patients.

Rheumatoid Factor and ANA
These are absent.

Radiology

Characteristic radiology changes may be seen at various sites:

SACROILIAC JOINTS

Radiological sacroiliitis is essential for the diagnosis of ankylosing spondylitis (Fig. 10.2).

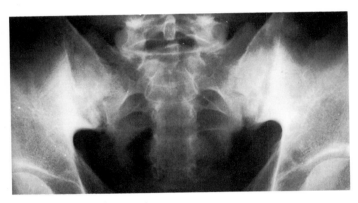

Fig. 10.2   X-ray of sacroiliac joints showing sacroiliitis.

Progressive changes include:
— sclerosis of the ilium and sacrum on either side of the joint
— haziness of the joint margins which later show erosions
— narrowing of the joint space which may progress to fusion
— when ankylosis is complete the periarticular sclerosis fades, sometimes leaving evidence of the previous joint line, known as a *ghost joint*.
Changes do not always progress through all stages.
Sacroiliitis is usually bilateral but may be unilateral or asymmetrical early in disease.

SPINE

Spinal changes include:
— 'squaring' of the vertebral bodies, i.e. loss of the normal anterior concavity on the lateral view
— syndesmosphyte formation, usually first seen at the thoracolumbar level
— apophyseal joint fusion, best seen in the cervical spine
— atlantoaxial subluxation
— calcification of the paraspinal ligaments.

In advanced disease:
— the characteristic 'bamboo spine' results from syndesmophyte or paraspinal ligament calcification around a normal disc space
— spondylodiscitis may develop in the lower thoracic or upper lumbar segments: erosive changes occur in anterior vertebral bodies adjacent to the disc which becomes progressively destroyed; angulation of the spine may occur. The appearance may resemble infection or trauma but is probably part of the spondylitic process.

LIGAMENTOUS ATTACHMENTS

Sites of ligamentous attachment become roughened and calcified, with a fluffy or 'whiskered' appearance particularly around the ischial tuberosities, pelvic brim, greater and lesser trochanters. The iliolumbar ligament and other ligaments may calcify.

PERIPHERAL JOINTS

Peripheral joints, particularly the hips and shoulders may show erosive changes like rheumatoid arthritis but with a greater tendency to ankylosis.

Diagnosis

Minimal diagnostic criteria include:
— history of inflammatory back pain
— limitation of spinal movement in all three planes
— radiological sacroiliitis.
The diagnosis is strongly supported by:
— iritis
— limitation of chest expansion

— peripheral arthritis of typical distribution
— positive family history.

In distinguishing spondylitis from mechanical back pain, the points which strongly support inflammatory disease are:
— back pain with stiffness unrelieved by rest
— elevated ESR
— radiological sacroiliitis.

DIFFERENTIAL DIAGNOSIS

Differential diagnosis of radiological changes includes:
Causes of bilateral sacroiliitis:
— ankylosing spondylitis
— Reiter's syndrome
— inflammatory bowel disease
— psoriasis.
Causes of unilateral sacroiliitis:
— infective sacroiliitis, e.g. TB
— any cause of bilateral sacroiliitis.
Conditions which may resemble sacroiliitis:
— osteitis condensans ilii (Fig. 10.3): particularly occurs in

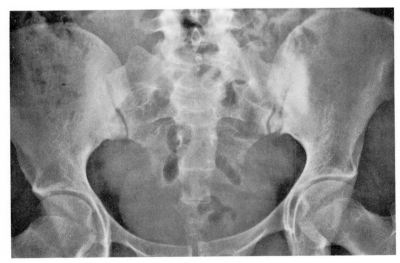

Fig. 10.3   Osteitis condensans ilii in a 24 year old woman who had borne three children. There is scleroisis on the iliac side of the sacroiliac joint. In this case, the left side is more severely affected than the right— usually the condition is more symmetrical. (Dr David Lewall, King Faisal Specialist Hospital, Saudi Arabia.)

multiparous women and appears as bony sclerosis adjacent to the sacroiliac joint on the ilial side without sacral sclerosis or erosive changes
— osteoarthritis of the sacroiliac joints: occurs in older patients with slight sclerosis of the joint margins and osteophyte formation at the lower edge of the anterior joint.

Conditions causing confusion with syndesmophytes:
— osteophytes of degenerative spinal disease
— senile ankylosing hyperostosis: occurs in older patients, with coarse calcification along the anterior vertebral bodies and across disc spaces; the sacroiliac joints are not involved.

Management

The major objectives of treatment are:
— the relief of pain and stiffness by use of medication
— the prevention of deformity by an exercise programme.
There are no drugs available which alter the course of the disease.

DRUG THERAPY

Drug treatment aims to control symptoms and thereby allow an effective physical therapy programme. The most useful drugs are:
— phenylbutazone at a dose of 200—600 mgm per day
— indomethacin capsules 25—50 mgm taken three or four times daily or as a suppository of 100 mgm at night
— other new N S A I D; aspirin is not generally useful.
A therapeutic trial of several agents may be necessary to find the most effective and best tolerated drug and dose for the individual patient. The withdrawal of phenylbutazone in many countries has left a gap in the management of ankylosing spondylitis patients.

Gold and penicillamine are not effective in treating the spinal disease. Sulphasalazine is reported to be useful in the treatment of the peripheral arthritis of alkylosing spondylitis.

PHYSICAL THERAPY

The aims of physical therapy are:
— to minimise spinal rigidity by mobilising exercises
— to ensure that, if ankylosis does occur, the spine is in a position of least flexion.
The programme should concentrate on:
— spinal extension exercises

— exercises to maintain mobility
— constant attention to posture to avoid spinal curvature
— the use of a firm, well-supported mattress and a low pillow
— avoidance of prolonged immobilisation
— deep breathing exercises
— avoidance of excessive spinal strain.

Swimming is an excellent form of recreational exercise.

Despite the apparent simplicity of the measures outlined, it is usually much harder to induce patients to undertake a regular exercise programme than to take tablets. The importance of the physical measures must be constantly reinforced and the programme supervised regularly.

SURGERY

Severe hip involvement may require total hip replacement which is often of great value but may be complicated by soft tissue calcification and ankylosis around the prosthesis.

Spinal ankylosis in a position of marked thoracic and cervical kyphosis can only be reversed by spinal osteotomy; the operation is not without considerable risk of cord damage and resultant paraplegia.

Spinal fractures require orthopaedic management.

OTHER MEASURES

Braces and spinal splinting have not generally been found effective in this disease, which may progress slowly over many years. The development of the patient's own spinal musculature is the best form of splinting.

Spinal irradiation relieves symptoms but does not alter the course of the disease. The ten-fold rise in the incidence of leukaemia following this form of therapy has led to its abandonment in most centres, though it is useful for local lesions in rare cases.

Course and prognosis

Ankylosing spondylitis shows a very wide range of severity. In some individuals, the disease is mild and although it may show periods of exacerbation with increased pain and stiffness, there is little permanent limitation of the spine.

At the other end of the spectrum, the disease may progress

relentlessly, causing marked and permanent spinal rigidity. Since patients with spinal pain tend to flex the back and neck, ankylosis occurs in this position producing variable degrees of a fixed C-shaped deformity, which at its most severe, is a disastrous functional position. Hip involvement is prognostically important, because it adds to the difficulty of mobility and further impairs function.

In early disease, there are no accurate guides to the course and likely outcome, other than the rate and degree of clinical progression.

REITER'S SYNDROME

Reiter's syndrome (R S) is defined as the combination of nonspecific urethritis, conjunctivitis, and arthritis. Incomplete forms of the syndrome are common. Reiter's syndrome is one form of *reactive arthritis*.

Epidemiology

Prevalence. Unknown; not rare. Less than 1% of patients with urethritis develop R S. Up to 20% of H L A-B27 patients with non-gonococcal urethritis may develop R S.

Sex. R S is male predominant but the ratio varies with the onset type:
— venereal   20:1 (male:female) see aetiology section.
— postdysenteric   10:1
— childhood   5:1

Age. 16–35 peak; R S occurs occasionally in childhood, occasionally in middle age.

Family history. Relatives have increased incidence of psoriasis, spondylitis and sacroiliitis.

Aetiology

Reiter's syndrome appears to be a good example of an inflammatory arthritis which is precipitated by an environmental agent in a genetically susceptible individual.

GENETIC FACTORS

Indicated by the HLA-B27 association (B27 is present in 60–80% of patients) and the familial aggregation with other seronegative arthropathies.

ENVIRONMENTAL FACTORS

Reiter's syndrome may occur following:

1   Sexually acquired non-specific urethritis
Frequently caused by *Chlamydia trachomatis* or ureaplasma urealyticum.
Note:
Because urethritis is an intrinsic feature of Reiter's syndrome, there has been a tendency to concentrate on a 'sexually acquired' aetiology.
2   Enteric infections
Particularly *Shigella flexneri*, *Yersinia entrocolitica*, or Salmonella.
3   Unknown factors.

While certain bacteria, especially some serotypes of *Shigella flexneri*, seem particularly arthritogenic in HLA-B27+ individuals, the mechanism of this interaction is unclear.

Pathology

ARTICULAR AND PERIARTICULAR

In early synovitis, there is intense hyperaemia with an infiltrate of lymphocytes and polymorphonuclear leucocytes and occasional surface necrosis which may resemble pyogenic synovitis. Later, chronic synovitis is often indistinguishable from rheumatoid arthritis. In addition there may be periostitis, particularly at the plantar surface of calcaneum and along the shafts of metatarsals and phalanges adjacent to inflamed joints. Other features include sacroiliitis and spondylitis.

MUCOCUTANEOUS

Skin lesions resemble pustular psoriasis while mucosal lesions are similar to skin lesions without hyperkeratosis.

Clinical features

ONSET

The onset is usually abrupt. Urethritis is usually the first symptom; conjunctivitis (often mild) may accompany or follow it. Arthritis begins 1–3 weeks after urethritis. Systemic illness, with fever, weight loss, and malaise is common.

UROLOGICAL LESIONS

Urethritis
Non-gonococcal, with mucoid or mucopurulent discharge, or dysuria.
Note:
Gonorrhoea and non-specific urethritis may be contracted simultaneously. Urethritis may occur in dysenteric Reiter's syndrome.

Prostatitis
Prostatitis and occasionally prostatic abscess.

Cystitis
Which may be haemorrhagic.

ARTICULAR LESIONS

Arthritis
— usually polyarticular and asymmetrical
— occasionally monoarticular
— predominantly lower limb especially knees and ankles
— sometimes severe with warm, tense, and very tender joints
— distribution often characteristic, e.g. interphalangeal joint of hallux, tarsometatarsal joints, M T P joints
— may become chronic and erosive.

Sausage digits (common)
— diffuse swelling of the whole digit especially a toe probably due to synovitis in the joints and tendon sheath; periostitis is often seen affecting metatarsal or phalanges (Fig. 10.4).

Achilles tendinitis (common)

Plantar fasciitis (common)
— may be severe
— fluffy calcaneal spur and periostitis along plantar surface of calcaneum often seen radiologically.

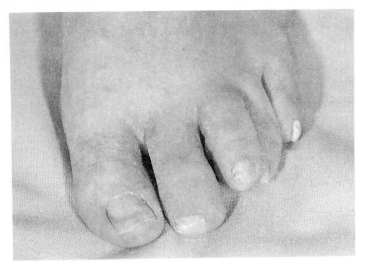

Fig. 10.4   Sausage digits in Reiter's syndrome.

Low back pain
— probably arising from sacroiliac joints
— is common early in the disease but generally settles after a few weeks.

Radiological sacroiliitis
— occurs in 20–40% of patients on long-term follow-up but it is often mild and asymmetrical.

Ankylosing spondylitis
— develops in approximately 10% of patients on long-term follow-up.

EYE LESIONS

Conjunctivitis
— usually mild
— often asymptomatic
— often settles in 1–4 weeks.

Uveitis
— may be recurrent and severe
— occurs especially in association with chronic erosive disease and sacroiliitis.

Keratitis, episcleritis, optic neuritis
— occasionally reported.

MUCOCUTANEOUS LESIONS

Keratoderma blenorrhagica
— a hyperkeratotic lesion, histologically resembling pustular psoriasis, but occurring particularly on the soles, sometimes

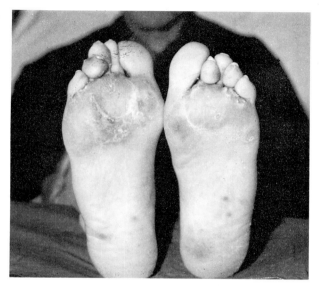

Fig. 10.5   Keratoderma blenorrhagica.

the palms, the glans penis, and occasionally becoming widespread
— nails become dystrophic with subungual hyperkeratosis.

Stomatitis
— small painless mouth ulcers
— very common
— often a recurring solitary feature in these patients and their relatives.

Circinate balanitis
— painless superficial coalescing ulcers around the glans penis.

OTHER VISCERAL LESIONS

Cardiac
— conduction defects
— aortic incompetence
— pericarditis.
Central nervous system
— involvement is very rare.

Laboratory tests

Haematology
Hb is usually normal early in disease but a normochromic normocytic anemia may develop.
Leucocytosis is common.
ESR may be > 100 mm/hr. Conversely, occasionally patients with very active arthritis have surprisingly normal ESRs.

HLA-B27
Present in 60–80%

Rheumatoid factor and ANA
These are absent

Synovial fluid:
Usually turbid, sometimes appears purulent.
WCC elevated, sometimes very high (50–100 000 mm^3), polymorphonuclear leucocytes predominate.
The complement level is usually high.

Radiology

During first attacks X-rays are usually normal. Later X-ray changes in Reiter's syndrome may include:
Juxta articular osteoporosis, joint space narrowing and erosions
Similar to those seen in rheumatoid arthritis but of different distribution.
— MTP joints asymmetrically affected
— interphalangeal of hallux
— calcaneal erosions at insertion of Achilles tendon.

Periostitis
— typically occurs contiguous to affected joints

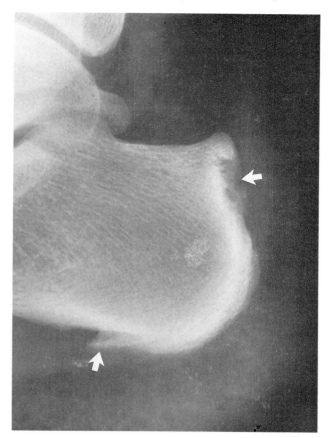

Fig. 10.6 The os calcis of a 20 year old man with Reiter's syndrome. There are erosions and a spur (arrows). Periosteal reaction in the phalanges, sacro-iliac joint erosions and juxta-articular osteoporosis are common. (Dr David Lewall, King Faisal Specialist Hospital, Saudi Arabia.)

— along metatarsals, phalanges of toes and fingers, and plantar surface of calcaneum.

Calcaneal spur
— typically soft and fluffy.

Sacroiliitis
— as in ankylosing spondylitis.

Spondylitis
—two types described
— identical to ankylosing spondylitis

— syndesmophytes which are larger, coarser, and less symmetrical than in typical ankylosing spondylitis.

The particular characteristics of Reiter's syndrome are erosive arthritis, predilection for the feet with relative sparing of the hands and periosteal changes.

Diagnosis

Reiter's syndrome is easily diagnosed when it presents with urethritis or diarrhoea followed by conjunctivitis and arthritis. Other presentations may cause more diagnostic difficulty:

ASYMMETRIC POLYARTHRITIS

Mild urethritis and conjunctivitis are easily overlooked unless specific enquiries are made; the presentation may appear to be arthritic.

The differential diagnosis usually includes:
— Reiter's syndrome
— psoriatic arthritis, where the pattern of joint involvement may be similar to Reiter's syndrome but the upper and lower limbs are equally affected and the sex incidence is equal
— seronegative rheumatoid arthritis, which is usually more symmetrical and has a female preponderance
— arthritis associated with infection or systemic disease.

MONOARTHRITIS

The arthritis of Reiter's syndrome may be severely inflammatory and, when monoarticular, the differential diagnosis must include:
— pyogenic arthritis
— crystal synovitis.
Joint aspiration with culture and examination of synovial fluid for bacteria and crystals is mandatory.

Other diseases, affecting both the joints and urogenital system, which may need to be distinguished include:

GONOCOCCAL ARTHRITIS

— since more than one venereal disease may be contracted simultaneously, gonococcal urethritis may occur with non-specific urethritis at the onset of Reiter's syndrome
— gonococcal polyarthritis is usually easily differentiated

clinically: there is a flitting arthritis or tenosynovitis, often at the wrist or ankle or knee, usually associated with fever, skin lesions or systemic malaise; females are affected more commonly than males.

BEHÇET'S SYNDROME

an uncommon disease characterised by:
— oral and genital ulceration
— uveitis
— skin lesions
— vascular lesions, including thrombophlebitis (Fig. 10.7)
— arthritis, often in a seronegative pattern
— other systemic lesions involving CNS and gastrointestinal tract.

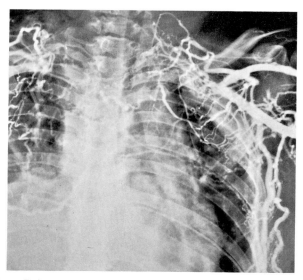

Fig. 10.7 Behçet's disease with thrombosis of the superior vena cava and both subclavian veins. Thrombosis and arterial aneurysm formation are established clinical features seen in a minority of patients with Behçet's. (Dr David Lewall, King Faisal Specialist Hospital, Saudi Arabia.)

Management

There is no specific treatment for Reiter's syndrome. In the future it should become possible to identify individuals who are particularly at risk and to shield them from the environmental triggering agents but, at present, effective predictive and preventive measures are not available.

URETHRITIS

Antibiotics have not been shown to influence the course of Reiter's syndrome or to affect the arthritis.

It is usual to treat non-specific urethritis in patients and their partners with appropriate antibiotics.

Other urological lesions may require specialist assessment.

EYE LESIONS

Conjunctivitis is mild and transient and usually requires no specific treatment. Iritis and more severe or prolonged conjunctivitis require expert ophthalmological treatment.

ARTHRITIS

Physical measures
— rest with splinting in an optimal position for acutely inflamed joints
— physiotherapy to relieve pain and stiffness
— an exercise programme to prevent muscle wasting, especially the quadriceps, and to maintain joint mobility.

Drug therapy
— the principal drugs used are indomethacin or phenylbutazone and local corticosteroid injections
— local corticosteroid injections are useful in treatment of plantar fasciitis, Achilles tendinitis, and persistent monoarthritis. Systemic corticosteroids are rarely indicated
— anti-rheumatic drugs; gold and penicillamine are generally ineffectual
— immunosuppressives have been reported to be effective in chronic arthritis and severe keratoderma blenorrhagica; most widely used at present is methotrexate.

Course and prognosis

Careful long-term patient follow-up has clearly revealed that Reiter's syndrome is not generally the benign self-limiting disease it was once considered.

Average episodes last 2–4 months but occasionally the arthritis becomes chronic from the outset.

Remissions may last for many years.

Recurrences occur in at least 50% of patients
— only about 50% of these are clearly preceded by non-specific urethritis or diarrhoea
— the pattern of recurrence may be the same as the initial attack but is often 'incomplete'.

Residual disability occurs in up to 30% of patients. Major problems include:
— painful, deformed feet
— visual impairment following recurrent uveitis
— cardiac lesions, e.g. aortic incompetence
— spinal involvement.

Long-term follow-up shows radiological sacroiliitis in 20–40% and ankylosing spondylitis in 10% of patients.

PSORIATIC ARTHRITIS

Once considered a variant of rheumatoid arthritis, psoriatic arthritis is currently held to be a real and distinct entity. Since five different but sometimes overlapping patterns of arthritis are recognised in this condition, the relationship between the skin and the joint disease appears to be a complex one.

Epidemiology

Prevalence About 1% of the population suffers from psoriasis and about 5% of patients with psoriasis develop arthritis. Thus about 0.05% of the population suffers psoriatic arthritis.

Sex The male: female ratio is equal.

Age Psoriatic arthritis most commonly occurs in the 30–50 age range, but occasionally in childhood.

Family history Both psoriasis and psoriatic arthritis are familial. Among the relatives of patients with psoriatic arthritis one study showed: 20% had psoriasis, 7% had sacroiliitis, 6% had uncomplicated seronegative arthritis, 6% had ankylosing spondylitis, 5% had psoriatic arthritis, and 1% had ulcerative colitis.

Aetiology

The aetiology of psoriatic arthritis is not known but it must inter-relate the pathogenic processes underlying both skin and synovial disease.

GENETIC FACTORS

Implicated by familial aggregation of psoriasis and psoriatic arthritis, and increased prevalence of H L A antigens B13, B17, B27, B38, B39 and Cw6 in psoriasis and psoriatic arthritis and of B27 in psoriatic spondylitis.

OTHER FACTORS

Streptococcal triggering of guttate psoriasis especially in children. Immunological mechanisms in psoriatic arthritis, where IgG rheumatoid factor is commonly present.
Abnormalities of skin metabolism and blood flow in psoriasis.

Pathology

ARTICULAR AND PERIARTICULAR

Synovitis histologically the same as in rheumatoid arthritis although bone resorption is sometimes prominent around affected joints. In addition there may be tenosynovitis, periostitis (as in Reiter's syndrome), and sacroiliitis and spondylitis.

Clinical features

SKIN AND NAIL CHANGES

Psoriatic skin lesions typically occur around the scalp and on the elbows and knees. Sometimes only a tiny patch is present in an easily overlooked site such as the hairline, umbilicus, natal cleft, or penis.
    Nail changes include multiple small pits, onycholysis (lifting

of the nail from its bed), and thickening of the nail with roughening and pigmentation.

ARTHRITIS

The onset is usually preceded by skin disease but may accompany or follow it. There is usually no correlation between activity of the psoriasis and activity of the arthritis.

Five patterns of arthritis are recognised in association with psoriasis but many patients show combinations of these.

DIP joint synovitis
— the most characteristic pattern of psoriatic arthritis
— often asymmetrical
— commonly associated with nail changes in the affected finger
— often associated with:

Asymmetric oligo- or monoarthritis
— commonest type
— generally mild
— 'sausage digit' results from involvement of the DIP and PIP joints with the flexor tendon sheath in the one finger or toe.

Rheumatoid-like arthritis
— seronegative
— indistinguishable from RA.

Arthritis mutilans
— rare
— very destructive arthritis with marked bone resorption around affected joints, causing deformities, e.g. 'opera glass hand'.

Ankylosing spondylitis
— occurs in 5–20% of patients with psoriatic arthritis.
Note:
Seropositive RA and psoriasis are both common diseases and they sometimes occur together.

EYE INVOLVEMENT

Conjunctivitis occurs in 20% of patients and iritis and episcleritis in 5% or less. Kerato conjunctivitis sicca (KCS) is rare.

Laboratory tests

Haematology
Hb may be low since normochromic normocytic anaemia usually accompanies extensive active synovitis; in patients with limited disease, the Hb may be normal.
ESR is often normal if synovitis is limited, but will be elevated with widespread active arthritis.

HLA antigens
HLA B13, B17, B27, B38, B39, and Cw6 are increased in psoriasis and psoriatic arthritis; some studies also report increased prevalence of DR4 and DR7.
HLA B27 is present in 15% of patients with peripheral arthritis and in 50–60% of patients with ankylosing spondylitis.

Rheumatoid factor and ANA
These are typically absent. IgG·rheumatoid factor is positive but this is not diagnostic.

Serum uric acid
Has been variously reported to be increased or normal in association with psoriasis.

Radiology

The X-ray changes in psoriatic arthritis include:

Erosive changes
— often identical to those seen in rheumatoid arthritis
— the distribution of changes may be diagnostically helpful
— a relative lack of osteoporosis around affected joints has been noted
— bony ankylosis tends to be more frequent than in RA.

Erosion
— seen at the tip of the terminal phalanges, especially in the hallux (acro-osteolysis).

Periostitis
— may occur along small bones adjacent to affected joints.

Bone resorption
— may be prominent. A 'pencil and cup' appearance is caused by 'whittling' of the distal ends of one bone and 'splaying' of the proximal end of the distal bone (Fig. 10.8).

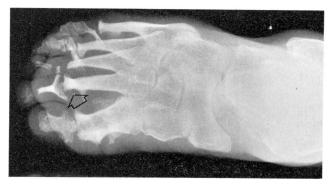

Fig. 10.8 Mutilating arthritis in a man with psoriasis. There is bone resorption in the metatarsals and phalanges and characteristic 'pencil-in-cup' deformity (arrow).

Sacroiliitis
— as in ankylosing spondylitis.

Spondylitis
— as in Reiter's syndrome, psoriatic spondylitis often shows syndesmophytes which are larger, coarser and less symmetrical than in typical ankylosing spondylitis.

Diagnosis

The combination of psoriasis and a seronegative inflammatory arthritis usually provides a sufficient basis for diagnosis. Diagnostic confusion may occur when the arthritis develops before the skin disease:

— it is well recognised that some patients with 'seronegative rheumatoid arthritis' will ultimately develop psoriasis

— occasionally patients present with an oligoarticular synovitis typical of psoriatic arthritis but without evidence of skin disease or nail changes; the diagnostic classification of these patients remains unsatisfactory.

Management

Psoriatic arthritis is managed in the same way as rheumatoid arthritis.

The peripheral arthritis often responds well to treatment with non-steroidal anti-inflammatory drugs or, when only a few joints are involved, to local steroid therapy. If these measures fail to control disease activity an anti-rheumatic drug is indicated. Gold is effective, is not associated with worsening of the psoriasis, and causes no more mucocutaneous toxicity than in rheumatoid arthritis. Immunosuppressive agents, particularly methotrexate, have been used to treat patients with severe skin or joint disease.

Psoriatic spondylitis is managed in the same way as ankylosing spondylitis.

Course and prognosis

The prognosis of psoriatic arthritis relates to the clinical type.

D I P arthritis and the oligoarticular type have a good prognosis with respect to function.

The rheumatoid-like type is usually milder and more episodic than seropositive rheumatoid arthritis.

Arthritis mutilans, as the name suggests, is severely destructive, responds poorly to treatment, but is fortunately rare.

Psoriatic spondylitis may run a course indistinguishable from ankylosing spondylitis.

ARTHROPATHIES OF INFLAMMATORY BOWEL DISEASE

Patients with ulcerative colitis and Crohn's disease may develop enteropathic arthritis, sacroiliitis, ankylosing spondylitis, and rarely hypertrophic osteoarthropathy associated with finger clubbing. Apart from some minor differences in prevalence, the arthropathies of ulcerative colitis and Crohn's disease can be regarded as identical.

ENTEROPATHIC ARTHRITIS

Enteropathic arthritis is a seronegative, non-erosive, typically oligoarticular synovitis related to the underlying inflammatory bowel disease. The aetiology is unknown but the synovitis may occur in response to bacterial antigens which have passed through damaged gut wall.

Epidemiology

Prevalence   It affects about 10% of patients with ulcerative colitis and 15–20% of patients with Crohn's disease.

Sex The male:female ratio is approximately equal.

Age Onset is variable but is most commonly in the 20–45 range.

Clinical features

ARTHRITIS

— usually of acute onset
— typically oligoarticular and often migratory
— non-deforming
— usually affects knee or ankle, but also wrists, hands and feet
— erythema nodosum sometimes accompanies arthritis
— course is usually self-limiting (less than 3 months duration in 60% of patients, more than 12 months duration in 10% of patients).

Relation to bowel disease
— arthritis usually follows onset of bowel disease
— arthritis is often but not invariably related to the activity of the bowel disease
— eradication of inflammatory bowel disease (e.g. by colectomy in ulcerative colitis) usually cures the arthritis.

Laboratory tests

Haematology
Anaemia and elevated E S R usually accompany inflammatory bowel disease.

Rheumatoid factor and ANA
These are usually absent.

HLA-B27
Shows no increase in frequency.

Synovial fluid
Inflammatory. W C C 2000–50 000/mm^3, predominantly polymorphonuclear leucocytes.

Diagnosis

Since only about 10% of patients develop this uncommon form of arthritis prior to the bowel disease, a good history usually allows a correct diagnosis. The type and pattern of joint involvement may need to be distinguished from other seronegative arthropathies such as peripheral onset of ankylosing spondylitis, Reiter's syndrome, and psoriatic arthritis, also from seronegative rheumatoid arthritis.

Arthritis and bowel disease is also seen in Whipple's disease (*see* p. 282).

Management

Control underlying inflammatory bowel disease.
Conservative measures
— rest
— physical therapy
— non-steroidal anti-inflammatory drugs, avoiding drugs which worsen the bowel disease.

SPONDYLITIS AND BOWEL DISEASE

Sacroiliitis and ankylosing spondylitis show a higher than expected prevalence in patients with ulcerative colitis and Crohn's disease although they do not appear causally related. The onset, severity, and progression of the spinal disease bears no constant relation to the activity or extent of the bowel disease. It is therefore assumed that ankylosing spondylitis and inflammatory bowel disease simply occur together more commonly than expected, possibly because some genetic factors predispose to the development of both disorders.

Clinical features

Ankylosing spondylitis occurring in association with inflammatory bowel disease is identical to uncomplicated ankylosing spondylitis except that
— the sex incidence is more nearly equal (male:female 1–2: 1)
— H L A-B27 is present in only about 60% of patients.

Management

Management is the same as for uncomplicated ankylosing spondylitis although special care must be taken in using non-steroidal anti-inflammatory drugs to avoid exacerbating the inflammatory bowel disease.

11 Juvenile Chronic Arthritis (Still's Disease)

Juvenile chronic arthritis (J CA) refers to an inflammatory arthritis of at least 3 months duration beginning in children less than 16 years of age, and excludes other recognisable rheumatic diseases such as those listed in the section on differential diagnosis (p. 122).

The terminology of childhood arthritis is confusing: juvenile chronic arthritis has also been called juvenile rheumatoid arthritis (J R A) in the U S A and Still's disease in the U K.

DISEASE SUBGROUPS

Juvenile chronic arthritis is not a single entity; it includes several subgroups, some of which may be recognised ultimately as quite separate diseases. Currently the classification of J CA subgroups is based on the mode of onset. Since some children only reveal the true pattern of their disease after months or years and others show changing characteristics which move them from one subgroup to another, the present system must be considered provisional. However, for so simple an approach it has proved a remarkably useful starting point for clinical, serological and immunogenetic studies. The major subgroups and their approximate frequency in J CA are given in Table 11.1.

Systemic onset refers to the presence of a persistent fever of

Table 11.1 Major subgroups and frequency of occurence in J CA

Subgroup	Frequency (%)
Systemic onset	10–20
Polyarticular:	
seronegative	20–30
seropositive	10–15
Pauciarticular:	40–50

Table 11.2 The clinical, serological and prognostic features of the major subgroups of JCA

	Systemic onset	Polyarticular		Pauciarticular	
		Seronegative	Seropositive	Early onset	Late onset
Sex ratio	M≥F	F>M	F>M	F>M	M>F
Age range (median)	Any age (4 years)	Any age	Late childhood (12 years)	Early childhood (3 years)	Late childhood (13 years)
Joints affected	Any joints Symmetric Peripheral	Any Joints Symmetric Peripheral	Any joints Symmetric Peripheral	Large joints Asymmetric	Large joints Asymmetric Lower limb
Other features	Fever Rash Lymphadenopathy Serositis	Lymphadenopathy	Nodules	Chronic uveitis	Acute uveitis
Serology	RF− ANA±	RF− ANA+20%	RF+100% ANA+60-75%	RF− ANA+50-90%	RF− ANA−
HLA association	?HLA Bw35 ?HLA DR4	?	HLA DR4	HLA DR5 HLA DR8	HLA B27
Prognosis	Severe arthritis in 20-25%	Severe arthritis in 10-15%	Progressive disease in 50%	Severe arthritis uncommon Visual impairment in 20% with chronic uveitis	Some develop ankylosing spondylitis

intermittent type with another characteristic feature, e.g. rash, lymphadenopathy, hepatosplenomegaly, pericarditis. Polyarticular arthritis refers to involvement of five joints or more. Pauciarticular arthritis refers to involvement of four joints or less. The clinical, serological and prognostic features of these subgroups are detailed in Table 11.2.

EPIDEMIOLOGY

Prevalence It is estimated that JCA affects approximately 1:1500 children.

Age of onset The typical age of onset varies in different subgroups; the most common age of presentation is in children under 5 years of age and it is unusual in children less than 6 months of age.

Sex ratio Overall, females are affected more often than males but the ratio varies in different subgroups.

AETIOLOGY

The aetiology of JCA is unknown. HLA antigen associations suggest genetic predisposition. Immunological abnormalities are considered important but remain poorly defined. Infectious agents of various types have been suspected and investigated but never incriminated.

PATHOLOGY

The synovial histology seen in all types of JCA may show changes identical to those of rheumatoid arthritis and other seronegative arthropathies. Nodules occurring in seropositive disease are histologically identical to those of adult rheumatoid arthritis. Nodules which occur rarely in seronegative polyarthritis histologically resemble those of rheumatic fever. The rash of systemic onset disease results from a mild mononuclear infiltrate around capillaries and venules but immunofluorescence is negative.

GENERAL CLINICAL FEATURES

The clinical and laboratory characteristics of the recognised subgroups of JCA are described separately. However, there are three important aspects in which J CA differs from arthritis in adults.

Arthritis

In children, complaints of pain and stiffness are often absent and the presentation may be impaired function, e.g. a limp, difficulty handling cutlery or turning off taps.

Inflammatory arthritis, rapidly causes muscle wasting and deformity
— fixed contractures at the elbow, wrist, hips and knees are common and develop quickly
— varus and valgus deformities may occur at the knees and ankles.

Bony ankylosis is more common than in adults.

Growth disturbances

Because chronic inflammatory arthritis causes prominent systemic effects and occurs at areas of very active growth, J CA may cause:
— generalised impairment of growth with delay of sexual maturation especially in systemic onset J CA
— localised growth disturbances due to overgrowth of epiphyses followed by premature epiphyseal fusion, both defects resulting from increased vascularity associated with inflammation. Also evident particularly in pauciarticular disease
— iatrogenic growth disturbances, e.g. vertebral collapse, resulting from administration of corticosteroids.

Eye involvement

Two types of eye involvement (*uveitis*), are seen.

CHRONIC UVEITIS

Chronic uveitis occurs particularly but not exclusively in patients with early onset pauciarticular J CA and postive A N A where it may be the presenting feature.

Clinical features
— insidious onset
— painless

— minimal signs until well advanced, when distortion of the pupil may be evident
— both eyes affected in 60%
— may precede or follow arthritis.
Often detected only on slit lamp examination.

Major effects
— keratatic precipitates in the anterior chamber
— posterior synechiae between the lens and iris
— band keratopathy: an opacity due to calcium deposition beneath the corneal epiphelium, extending across the cornea from the limbus
— secondary cataract formation
— glaucoma
— blindness.
It is mandatory that all patients with J C A have repeated ophthalmological examinations by slit lamp which may be the only means of detecting early disease.

ACUTE UVEITIS

Acute uveitis occurs particularly in older boys with lower limb arthritis plus a minor sacroiliitis and H L A B27.

Clinical features
— acute painful red eye
A better prognosis than chronic iritis.

CLINICAL AND LABORATORY FEATURES OF SUBGROUPS

Systemic onset

SEX AND AGE

— usually afects more boys than girls
— typically in children under 5 but may occur later.

SYSTEMIC FEATURES

Fever:
— characteristic pattern with high daily spike in the afternoon or evening

— marked malaise, listlessness and irritability often accompany the fever but resolves as the temperature subsides.

Rash:
— often accompanies fever and is brought out by a warm bath or by pressure (Koebner effect)
— occurs on the limbs or trunk; less often on the face
— typically macular or maculopapular
— pink and nonpruritic
— variable size but usually less then 0.5 cm.

Lymphadenopathy:
— generalised
— may be marked.

Splenomegaly ± hepatomegaly:
— less common than lymphadenopathy
— serious hepatitis occurs in a minority.

Pericarditis ± pleurisy:
— occasionally pneumonitis and myocarditis occur.

Cerebral symptoms:
— drowsiness, meningism and even seizures may occur.

ARTHRITIS

Initially joint symptoms may be absent or arthralgia alone may be present.

Interval between the development of systemic symptoms and the onset of arthritis is variable. Arthritis is usually absent at onset but has developed in 50% by 3 months.

Arthritis is typically polyarticular and symmetrical, especially involving the wrists, carpi, knees, ankles and tarsi.

Flexor tenosynovitis may be prominent in the hands.

Arthritis may be identical to that seen in seronegative polyarticular J C A.

LABORATORY FEATURES

Leucocytosis is typical
— 20 000–50 000 mm³.
— predominantly polymorphonuclear leucocytes.

Thrombocytosis is common: often $> 500\,000\,mm^3$.

E S R usually high; often $> 100\,mm/hr$.

Anaemia, normochromic normocytic.

Rheumatoid factor is negative.

ANA usually negative.

Hypergammaglobulinaemia is common.

Liver function tests:
— elevation of liver enzymes may be seen particularly in association with high salicylate levels.

Proteinuria may be due to
— fever, orthostatic proteinuria, amyloidosis or drug therapy.

Seronegative polyarthritis

SEX AND AGE

Predominantly affects females (female:male, 9:1).

Occurs at any age.

ARTHRITIS

Onset sometimes acute but more often insidious.

Occasionally develops after a pauciarticular onset.

Typically affects knees, wrists, ankles and MCP, PIP and DIP joints.

Tenosynovitis may occur in the hands and feet.

Cervical spine is affected in 30% of cases.

Temporomandibular joint may also be involved (Fig. 11.1)

Hip and shoulder involvement occurs late.

EXTRA-ARTICULAR FEATURES

Extra-articular features may include:
— intermittent low grade fever
— lymphadenopathy
— splenomegaly and hepatomegaly are unusual
— chronic uveitis occurs in around 5%.

LABORATORY FEATURES

Elevated ESR, anaemia, leukocytotosis and thrombocytosis occur but are less marked than in systemic onset.

Rheumatoid factor is negative.

ANA positive in up to 25%.

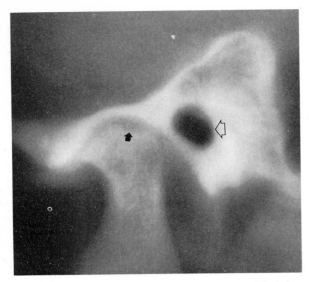

Fig. 11.1 Juvenile rheumatoid arthritis in a 19 year old. A lateral tomogram of the temporomandibular joint shows narrowing of the joint and erosion of the mandibular condyle (solid arrow). The open arrow points to the internal auditory canal. This is a common site of involvement in the juvenile form of rheumatoid arthritis. (Dr David Lewall, King Faisal Specialist Hospital, Saudi Arabia.)

Seropositive polyarthritis

SEX AND AGE

Predominantly affects girls and usually begins in later childhood, 10–15 years.

ARTHRITIS

Usually insidious onset, symmetrically involving the peripheral joints.

Often severe and progressive.

Especially affects the ulnar styloids, wrists, MCP, PIP joints, knees, ankles and MTP joints.

Tenosynovitis is common and tendon rupture may occur.

Hip involvement is common and may be severe.

X-ray changes occur early.

EXTRA-ARTICULAR FEATURES

Nodules are identical clinically and histologically to those which occur in adult rheumatoid arthritis.
Rheumatoid vasculitis may occur.

LABORATORY FEATURES

Anaemia and E S R are common.
Rheumatoid factor positive.
A N A is positive in 60–75%.
H L A-D R4, the antigen associated with adult rheumatoid arthritis is also found with increased frequency in seropositive J CA.

Pauciarticular—early onset

SEX AND AGE

Predominantly affects girls and
commonly affects children aged around 3 years.

ARTHRITIS

Usually asymmetrical.
Often affects the knees, ankles, elbows, wrists or a single finger with both P I P joint synovitis and tenosynovitis.
Some progress to polyarticular disease.

CHRONIC UVEITIS

Particularly common in the group of young children with pauciarticular arthritis and positive A N A.
May be present at the onset of arthritis or develop subsequently.

LABORATORY FEATURES

Anaemia and elevation of the E S R is typically less evident in this group.
Rheumatoid factor negative.
A N A positive 50–90%.
H L D-D R5 and D R8 are associated with early onset pauciarticular J CA with chronic uveitis and A N A.

Pauciarticular—late onset

SEX AND AGE

Predominantly affects boys, especially adolescents.

ARTHRITIS

Usually asymmetrical and predominantly lower limbs, especially involving the hips, knees and ankles.
Hip involvement may be severe.
On long term follow up, more than 50% develop sacroiliitis and some develop ankylosing spondylitis.

EXTRA-ARTICULAR FEATURES

Acute uveitis develops in 20–25%.
Rarely: aortic incompetence and inflammatory bowel disease.

LABORATORY FEATURES

Anaemia, elevated E S R may be present.
H L A-B27 typically positive in this group.

Pauciarticular—other

A variety of other less well characterised patterns have been recognised:
— persistent pauciarticular J C A without uveitis or A N A
— pauciarticular progressing to polyarticular disease, this subgroup includes some patients who also develop psoriasis
— monoarticular disease with negative rheumatoid factor and A N A and a good prognosis.

RADIOLOGICAL CHANGES

Early

Soft tissue swelling or periarticular osteoporosis.

Later

Changes may include:
1 Loss of joint space.

2   Irregularity of the joint surface with a 'crumpled' double contour appearance, particularly in the carpus; erosions are uncommon and occur late.

3   Periosteal new bone formation, particularly along the metacarpals, metatarsals and phalanges, contiguous with the affected joints.

4   Growth disturbances:
Accelerated growth at sites of inflammation may manifest as:
— premature development of ossification centres, e.g. in the carpus
— overgrowth of epiphyses
Premature epiphyseal closure.

5   Changes in the cervical spine:
— apophyseal joint fusion often initially at C2-3 levels: subsequently extending down the cervical spine
— vertebral body underdevelopment
— atlanto-axial subluxation; subluxation at other levels less common than in rheumatoid arthritis.

6   Bony fusion.

Characteristic changes in J C A subgroups

1   Seronegative polyarticular J C A:
— osteoporosis occurs early but other changes are not prominent until late.

2   Seropositive polyarticular J C A:
Severe changes may occur early:
— atlanto-axial subluxation
— severe hip damage with protrusio acetabuli.

3   Pauciarticular J C A:
— changes occur early especially in large joints
— growth disturbances often obvious
— sacroiliitis is common in older H L A-B27 positive patients.

DIAGNOSIS

The child presenting with musculoskeletal symptoms often constitutes a difficult diagnostic problem. Steps essential in reaching a correct diagnosis are:

1   Distinguish arthralgia and limb pain from arthritis. Pain, which is persistently unaccompanied by any objective changes,

ill-health, growth disturbances, or any laboratory abnormalities, is rarely due to a serious rheumatic disease.

2 Avoid premature diagnosis of JCA. It is impossible to reach a diagnosis of JCA confidently if the illness has been present for less than 3 months.

3 Obtain all possible diagnostic clues from the patient's past history and particularly the family history.

4 Consider the range of diagnostic possibilities suggested by the pattern of joint involvement (*see* next section).

DIFFERENTIAL DIAGNOSIS

Arthritis with fever and other systemic features

INFECTION

Viral:
— a number of viral infections cause fever and arthritis, often with a maculopapular rash.
— these include adenovirus, cytomegalo virus, hepatitis B infections, arbovirus, rubella, chickenpox, mumps, EB virus.

Bacterial:
— meningococcal and gonococcal bacteraemia (*see* Chap. 23)
— septicaemia may be accompanied by polyarthralgia or polyarthritis.

Mycoplasmal:
— M.pneumoniae may provoke a Stevens-Johnson syndrome with fever, mucocutaneous lesions and arthritis.
— Lyme arthritis due to a spirochaete causes fever, arthritis and erythema chronicum migrans.

POST-INFECTIVE ARTHRITIS

Rheumatic fever
Features which favour JCA:
— onset under five years
— non-migratory polyarthritis
— neck involvement
— typical rash
— remittent fever.
Features common to both JCA and rheumatic fever:
— asymmetrical polyarthritis

— elevated A S O T
— pericarditis
— response to salicylates.

Reactive arthritis following:
— enteric infections with Shigella, Salmonella, Yersinia, Campylobacter
— sexually acquired infections.

LEUKAEMIA AND OTHER MALIGNANCY

Blood dyscrasias in children commonly present with articular features and may be readily confused with systemic onset JCA. Neuroblastoma may present with bone pain.

OTHER CONNECTIVE TISSUE DISEASES

SLE
Dermatomyositis
Arteritides including:
— Henoch-Schönlein purpura
— Kawasaki disease.

OTHER CONDITIONS

Familial Mediterranean fever.
Arthritis occurring with inflammatory bowel disease, drug reactions, acne conglobata.

Polyarthritis

Other seronegative arthropathies
Psoriatic arthritis
Enteropathic arthritis including coeliac disease
Reiter's syndrome.

Metabolic, developmental and other systemic diseases
Familial hypercholesterolemia
Scurvy
Farber's disease
Immunodeficiency
Hypertrophic osteoarthropathy
Mucopolysaccharidoses
Epiphyseal disorders.

Trauma
Battered baby.

Pauciarthritis

Other seronegative arthropathies
— psoriatic arthritis
— Reiter's syndrome
— enteropathic arthritis.

Hypo gammaglobulinaemia

Palindromic rheumatism

Gout (enzyme defects)

Monoarthritis

Infection
— tuberculosis
— bacterial

Trauma
— internal derangement.

Haemangioma and neoplasm

Vegetable (thorn) synovitis

MANAGEMENT

The course and prognosis in JCA is closely related to the onset subgroup. In the majority, the disease ultimately becomes inactive and the aim of management is to ensure that when that stage is reached the child has as few physical, educational and social limitations as possible.

The full co-operation of the parents is crucial to optimal management which may be long and difficult. The parents should be fully informed as to the nature of the disease and the aims of treatment.

Prevention of deformity and muscle wasting

REST

Essential but it must be combined with activity. While the disease is active, children require adequate rest at night and often additional rest periods during the day. Involvement of lower limb joints requires some modification of activity and the avoidance of contact sports and situations in which affected joints are likely to be damaged.

GENERAL MOBILITY

Must be maintained and the child should not be put to bed unless, as is sometimes the case during periods of systemic disease, it is essential.

JOINTS

Must be put through a full range of movement several times each day, preferably by active exercises or if necessary by gentle passive movement.

MUSCLES

Must be exercised and their power maintained; hydrotherapy is a very useful component of the physical therapy programme.

SPLINTING OF THE INVOLVED JOINTS

This includes:
Wrists: night rest splints and day work splints should maintain a slightly extended position.
Knees and ankles: POP night splints with the knees fully extended and the ankles at 90°.
Cervical spine: a collar to prevent fixed flexion during episodes of pain and active involvement.

GOOD POSTURE

When sitting and lying. A bed should have a firm surface and a low pillow. Correctly fitting footwear is also important.

Correction of deformity

Serial splinting of wrists and knees to correct position.
Prone lying or *hip traction* to correct flexion deformity.
Insoles or *T-strap and iron* to improve ankle position.
Orthopaedic procedures to correct problems too advanced for more conservative measures.

Suppression of disease activity—drug therapy

The principles are similar to those employed in adult disease.

NON-STEROIDAL ANTI-INFLAMMATORY DRUGS (NSAID)

Salicylates remain the drugs of first choice.
— the correct dose is one which maintains a serum salicylate level between 1–2 mmol/l and this is achieved with around 90 mgm/kg body weight/day in divided doses.
— side effects: children rarely complain of tinnitus and early overdose is often manifest as drowsiness or over-breathing; liver enzyme elevations are common in children with blood levels in excess of 2 mmol/l.

Although lagging behind adult practice, non-steroidal anti-inflammatory agents are gradually becoming more widely used in children. Some of the newer NSAID may be used with caution but phenylbutazone and its derivatives should be avoided.

ANTI-RHEUMATIC DRUGS

Gold and D-penicillamine have both been used and appear to be no more toxic in children than in adults.
Indications:
In seropositive JCA:
— early introduction is warranted because this type of disease is so commonly severe and progressive.
In seronegative JCA:
— severe and persistent disease despite optimal use of non-steroidal anti-inflammatory agents and a physical therapy programme
— patients on corticosteroids who require an anti-rheumatic drug to allow steroid dose reduction.

CORTICOSTEROIDS

Indications:
— severe systemic disease
— severe joint involvement which is progressing despite a full conservative regimen and an adequate trial of other anti-rheumatic drugs
— chronic iridocyclitis not controlled by local steroid therapy.

If steroids are used, an alternate day regimen should be employed since as little as 5 mg daily in children suppresses growth.

INTRA-ARTICULAR STEROIDS

These may be used for the control of single, persistently active joints but only after intercurrent infection has been excluded.

They are also useful in flexor tenosynovitis where hydrocortisone acetate rather than the longer acting preparations should be used.

Intra-articular steroids should be used with caution and injections of any one joint probably should not be repeated within a 12–24 month period.

IMMUNOSUPPRESSIVES

These are rarely warranted.

Amyloidosis, a potentially fatal complication, justifies their use.

Treatment of uveitis

Both acute and chronic uveitis require treatment with mydriatics and local corticosteroids. Chronic uveitis, which may be associated with the development of band keratopathy, cataracts and glaucoma, requires expert ophthalmological supervision.

Education and social support

Because the disease remains active and treatment must be continued for many years, it is essential that every effort is made to promote the education and normal socialisation of affected children.

During some phases of the illness, periods of prolonged hospitalisation may be necessary and this is best undertaken in centres equipped with facilities for hydrotherapy, physical therapy and schooling, so that disruption to the latter is minimised.

COMPLICATIONS

1 Amyloidosis. Variable frequency in different parts of the world, especially common in continental Europe but uncommon in the U S A and Australia.
2 Growth retardation and delay in sexual maturation.
3 Fractures.
4 Iatrogenic complications.

PROGNOSIS

The prognosis of J C A relates well to the onset subgroup.

SYSTEMIC ONSET

Around 50% of children will go into remission over five years
— the remainder show periods of remission and relapse and in the majority the disease is dominated by polyarticular arthritis which is severe in about half of them
— death may occur as a result of early infection or the late development of amyloidosis.

SERONEGATIVE POLYARTHRITIS

Arthritis often persists over many years but is severe in a minority.

SEROPOSITIVE POLYARTHRITIS

This group has the most severe disease and hence the worst prognosis
— severe arthritis occurs in about 50%.

PAUCIARTICULAR DISEASE

Severe arthritis is uncommon although growth disturbances cause deformities
— some patients, from late onset pauciarticular group, will develop ankylosing spondylitis or severe hip disease

— chronic iritis may be a serious problem in early onset ANA positive JCA and around 20% of those will suffer some impairment of visual acuity with blindness occurring in a minority.

Overall, 70–80% of children make a satisfactory recovery without serious functional impairment. At 15 year follow-up, more than 80% of a group of children with JCA were able to work.

12 Systemic Lupus Erythematosus

Systemic lupus erythematosus (SLE, lupus) is a multisystem disorder predominantly affecting young women and characterised by widespread organ involvement, a profound immunological disturbance, and a tendency to exacerbation and remission.

EPIDEMIOLOGY

Prevalance During the past 20 years, SLE has emerged as a major cause of inflammatory arthritis. Whether there has been a real increase in prevalence, or whether the increase simply reflects the recognition of milder cases is uncertain. In some studies (e.g. from California and the West Indies) up to 1 in 250 females have been affected. In certain Far East countries, the prevalence of SLE may exceed that of RA.

Geography SLE is worldwide, though in some areas such as the West Indies, Singapore and the Far East, it appears to be particularly common and is probably commoner in sunnier countries.

Sex The female:male ratio is 9:1 (in childbearing years the female predominance may be even higher).

Age at onset Usually 10–35 and is commonest in early 20s.

Family history Very slight increase of SLE (and of other autoimmune diseases) has been shown in family members of SLE patients.

AETIOLOGY

As with most of the rheumatic diseases, the cause is unknown, though environmental, genetic, and hormonal factors are implicated. The evidence for these is summarised as follows:

INFECTIVE

— clinical features in the acute stage (fever, lymphadenopathy, leukopenia) suggest 'viral' illness
— a lupus-like disease occurring in a species of dog can be transmitted by cell-free spleen extracts to normal recipient animals
— C-type virus antigens are implicated in the lupus-like disease of New Zealand B/W F_1 mice
— lymphocytotoxic antibodies (often seen following certain acute viral infections) are seen not only in 80% of SLE patients, but in up to 50% of their household contacts.

GENETIC

— increased familial tendency
— twin studies suggest genetic tendency
— animal studies—disease expression under genetic control
— individuals with genetic complement deficiencies have a markedly increased tendency to develop SLE
— individuals with chronic biological false-positive tests for syphilis (genetic tendency) have an increased susceptibility to SLE and lupus-like syndromes
— HLA studies suggest increase HLA-A1, B8, DR3 and C4 null allele association in certain countries.

HORMONAL

— female predominance
— premenstrual exacerbations common
— exacerbations common in puerperium
— increased incidence in Klinefelter's syndrome
— tendency to flare on oral contraceptives in occasional patients
— preliminary evidence of abnormal oestrogen metabolism in males with SLE.

UV LIGHT

— tendency to disease flare in sunlight (in approximately 50% of patients)
— DNA after UV irradiation becomes immunogenic.

DRUGS

There is little to suggest that drug LE is related to true SLE (hydralazine LE for example is related to HLA D4 while SLE is not). However, in patients with SLE or a lupus 'diathesis', certain drugs such as sulphonamides may exacerbate the disease.

IMMUNOLOGICAL

Although the immunopathological findings in SLE may not be the 'cause' of the disease, they clearly play a major role and are summarised here.

Impaired suppressor T cell function
Many different studies have shown that, during disease exacerbation (and *probably* also in remission), suppressor cell function is impaired. One of the sequelae of this is:

Overproduction of antibodies by B cells
A wide variety of antibodies (including antinuclear, antilymphocyte and antiviral) is produced. Interestingly, organ-specific autoantibodies do not seem to be excessively common. This overproduction of autoantibodies contributes to:

Direct damage
e.g. Coombs'-positive haemolytic anaemia, antibody mediated thrombocytopenia.

Indirect damage
Through the formation of antigen-antibody complexes (either 'in situ' or circulating).

PATHOLOGY

The predominant lesions are:
— fibrinoid necrosis
— haematoxylin bodies
— immune complex deposition.

FIBRINOID NECROSIS

An eosinophilic acellular necrotic material, usually surrounded by an inflammatory reaction; found in smaller blood vessels (arterioles, venules and capillaries) and on membranes such as pleura and joint capsules.

HAEMATOXYLIN BODIES

Altered nuclear material—the counterpart of the L E cell.

IMMUNE COMPLEX DEPOSITION

Evidence of immune complex deposition (consisting of deposits of immunoglobulin and complement in kidney (glomeruli), skin (dermal-epidermal junction), blood vessels, and occasionally elsewhere. On light and fluorescent microscopy, these are demonstable as lumpy or irregular deposits. Electron microscopy shows them to be electron-dense.

Other principal pathological changes

SKIN

Discoid
Follicular plugging and scarring.

S L E
Very little on light microscopy, but in up to 80% of biopsies of affected skin, fluorescence shows a 'band' of immune complex at the dermal-epidermal junction.

KIDNEYS

Immune complex deposition.
Focal or diffuse glomerulonephritis.
Crescents in severe cases.
Fibrinoid necrosis of arterioles or arteries.

CNS

Microinfarcts.
Venous thrombosis.
Choroid plexus immune complexes.

HEART

Pericarditis (the commonest lesion).
Myocarditis.
Libman–Sacks endocarditis. A now rare complication of severe S L E consisting of non-infective verrucous endocarditis.
Pulmonary hypertension.

BLOOD VESSELS

Mainly arterioles and capillaries affected.
Fibrinoid necrosis.
Thrombophlebitis.

SPLEEN

'Onion skin' thickening (concentric layers of fibrosis around the splenic arterioles, Fig. 12.1). is almost pathognomonic for SLE.

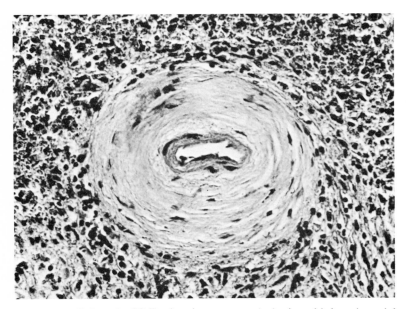

Fig. 12.1   Spleen in SLE, showing concentric 'onion-skin' periarterial fibrosis. (H&E × 340. Dr. Shirley Amin, University Hospital of the West Indies.)

JOINTS

Fibrinoid deposition.

LUNGS AND PLEURA

Pleural adhesions and effusion.
Interstitial pneumonitis (rare).

Recurrent atelectasis.
Infections.

CLINICAL FEATURES

S L E may affect almost any organ system in the body (the liver being notably rarely affected). The commonest presentation is arthralgia and skin rash in young women. The disease has a marked tendency to exacerbation and remission.

General features

Table 12.1 lists the commoner clinical manifestations of S L E. During disease flares, there may be general malaise, accompanied

Table 12.1 Major clinical manifestation of SLE in 150 patients. (From Estes and Christian (1971) *Medicine* **50**, 85.)

Manifestation	%
Musculo-articular	95
Cutaneous	81
Fever	77
Neuropsychiatric	59
Renal	53
Pulmonary	48
Cardiac	38

by arthralgias, rashes, fever (sometimes high and 'swinging'), depression, and headache. There is often a past history of drug allergies, arthralgia or pleurisy. Important features of the disease are livedo reticularis and variable alopecia.

SKIN

Almost any form of skin lesion may occur. The major skin manifestations of S L E are:
Vasculitis
In various forms, particularly livedo reticularis, fingertip (subungal) infarcts (Fig. 12.2), and vasculitic lesions on the elbows, soles of the feet, and palms.

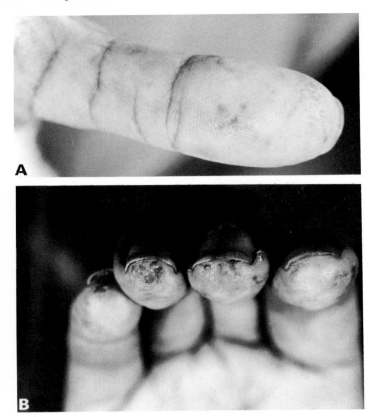

Fig. 12.2 A, B.   Digital vasculitis and finger tip infarction in S L E.

'Butterfly' facial rash (or 'blush')
Present in approximately 50% of patients at some stage.
Photosensitivity.
Sensitivity to U V light is variable and generally more marked
during active disease.
Alopecia.
Present in over 60% of patients. Usually patchy. Occasionally
accompanied by new hair growth on forehead.
Note:
In discoid L E, alopecia may be prominent, severe and scarring.
Others.
Mouth ulcers, purpura, urticaria, thrombophlebitis (may antedate
the diagnosis of S L E by months or years). Raynaud's pheno-

menon (usually mild to moderate. Severe Raynaud's more typical of mixed connective tissue disease).

MUSCULOSKELETAL

Joint pains occur in most SLE patients but *erosive* arthritis is exceptionally rare.
Tendon lesions (especially contractures) are prominent (Fig. 12.3).
Aseptic necrosis (almost always related to steroid therapy).
Myositis occurs in 10–30%, but is usually mild.

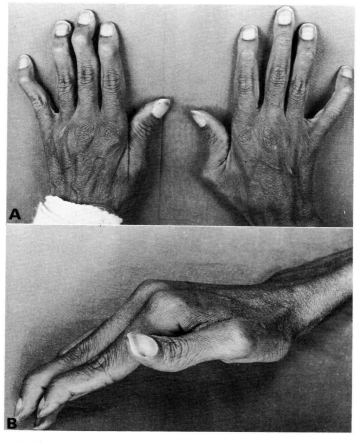

Fig. 12.3A, B.   Mild deforming arthritis in SLE.

VASCULAR

Clinical evidence of vasculitis includes:
— cutaneous vasculitis (*see above*)
— thrombophlebitis
— retinal vasculitis (demonstrated on fluorescein angiography or, in florid cases, seen clinically as cytoid bodies).

Note:
'Large' vessel vasculitic lesions or infarction of organs is unusual

HEART

Pericarditis occurs in 30–50%. Effusions are usually small and tamponade is rare.
Myocarditis is common in mild form but rarely presents major clinical problems.
'Libman–Sacks' endocarditis is very rare—the diagnosis is usually made in clinicopathological conferences, but rarely in clinical practice.
Recently, a number of patients, notably those with thrombotic tendencies, have been noted to develop pulmonary hypertension.

LUNG

Routine lung function testing in S L E reveals abnormalities in up to 80% (commonly a mixture of restrictive and diffusion defects). However, as distinct from scleroderma, major pulmonary involvement is rare.
The commonest problem is recurrent pleurisy and pleuritic pain (present in over 60%).
In a small number of patients, diaphragmatic weakness contributes to 'shrinking lungs' (Fig. 12.4).

RETICULO-ENDOTHELIAL SYSTEM

Splenomegaly (rarely massive) occurs in 25% and lymphadenopathy in 50%. Sophisticated studies have suggested that impaired R E S function might contribute to the excess circulating immune complexes seen in S L E.

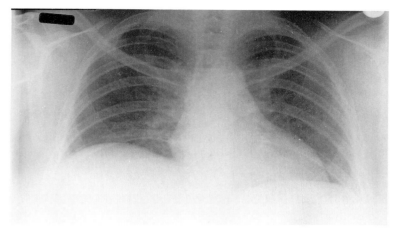

Fig. 12.4 'Shrinking lungs' in SLE. This severe form of lung disease in SLE appears to be predominantly due to progressive elevation of the diaphragm.

BLOOD

Haematological abnormalities are present at some stage in the majority of S L E patients.

Red cells
Normochromic, normocytic ('inflammatory') anaemia occurs in 75%.
Coombs-positive haemolytic anaemia 10–20%.

White cells
Low total white cell counts are an important clinical feature in S L E. Lymphopenia is the commonest abnormality, occurring in 65%, though neutropenia (under 1000 per mm^3) occurs in 10–20%.

Platelets
Platelet abnormalities play an important, though ill-understood, part in the widespread vasculitis of S L E. Mild thrombocytopenia is common; more severe thrombocytopenia is unusual (10%), but many precede the diagnosis by years.

Clotting factors
A variety of antibodies against various clotting factors have been described in S L E. Of these, the most important is the lupus anticoagulant, an antibody directed against prothrombin activa-

tor. This antibody is also clinically associated with 'false-positive' serology for syphilis. However, it is rarely associated with an increased bleeding tendency—in fact it is now known to be associated with an increased tendency to *clotting* problems (especially deep vein thrombosis and pulmonary embolus) in S L E.

KIDNEY

Clinical renal involvement (abnormal urinary sediment, abnormal renal function tests) occurs in some 50% of patients, though with the recognition of milder cases of S L E, the percentage with significant renal disease may fall. The most common clinical feature is proteinuria. Hypertension is an unusual presentation of S L E. The main types of renal involvement in S L E are summarised in Table 12.2.

Kidney biopsy is usually performed as a 'baseline' procedure only in patients with clinical evidence of renal disease.

Table 12.2   Kidney involvement in S L E

Involvement	Pathology	Clinical features
Focal proliferative	Segmental proliferation of glomeruli	Proteinuria Prognosis usually good Progression to diffuse proliferative rare Many regress
Diffuse proliferative	Proliferation in most glomeruli Crescents and sclerosis in most severe cases	Proteinuria Casts Renal failure Hypertension Remission *may* occur with treatment
Membranous	Finely granular deposits of immuno-globulin Immunofluorescent staining may appear linear	Proteinuria Nephrotic syndrome Good response in most cases to treatment
Mesangial	Mesangial hypercellularity and deposits of immune complexes	May remain 'subclinical' Usually benign

NERVOUS SYSTEM (Table 12.3)

Neuropsychiatric features are prominent in SLE. Particularly common are episodes of depression and behavioural problems which are not related to therapy and usually resolve spontaneously. The higher percentage of seizures or cerebrovascular accidents reported in older series is probably due to a failure to recognise the more subtle and common neuropsychiatric abnormalities. Epileptic seizures are not only common in SLE but may antedate the diagnosis by many years.

Table 12.3 Principal CNS involvement in SLE

Symptoms	Features
Headaches	May be migrainous
Depression	Occurs in up to 60% patients
Psychosis	Often reversed by steroid therapy
Behavioural problems	Vary from subtle to gross
Seizures	Include petit mal. May occur years before diagnosis
Paraplegia	Myelitis and Guillain-Barre syndrome may occur
Hemiplegia	Rare. Associated with the lupus anticoagulant
Cranial nerve lesions	Rare
Chorea	And other movement disorders (may also occur during pregnancy in SLE)
Meningitis	Lymphocytic
Peripheral neuropathy	Uncommon (less than 10% of patients)

Aetiology of CNS Involvement
Vascular
— widespread cerebral vasculitis is a factor in some cases. Possibly more important is a tendency to widespread venous thrombosis.
Immune complex deposition
— seen in the choroid plexus.
Other
— certain lymphocytotoxic antibodies cross-react with brain antigens. IgG antineuronal antibodies have been demonstrated in some patients.

Investigation of CNS disease
There is a disappointing lack of investigative aids, but the following should be considered:

EEG
— diffuse abnormalities seen in most patients.

Brain scan
— fluctuating abnormalities in a minority.

Oxygen scan
— inhalation of labelled oxygen provides a scan of cerebral tissue (under assessment).

NMR scan
— very restricted availability but useful for demonstrating cerebral infarction.

CAT scan
— useful for demonstrating cerebral infaction but unhelpful in milder cases.

CSF analysis
— useful if infection is suspected; otherwise changes are nonspecific with elevation of protein and cell count.

CSF C4
— low in a small number with florid CNS lupus. In practice not a useful investigation.

Retinal angiography
— may demonstrate leakage of dye in retinal vasculitis. Correlates poorly with clinical features.

Infection

Infections are commoner in active SLE, over and above those related to therapy with steroids and immunosuppressives. However it is doubtful whether mild SLE *per se* predisposes to infections. Tuberculosis may present particular diagnostic difficulties in the SLE patient on corticosteroid therapy.

SLE and pregnancy

Pregnancy is not contraindicated, even where mild renal involvement is present.
There is no apparent long-term effect on the mother.
There is a tendency to increased SLE activity in puerperium.
There is a higher incidence of spontaneous abortion.

There is a slightly raised incidence of congenital heart block in infants born of mothers with active S L E.

Drug-induced lupus

This is a rare syndrome (far less common than idiopathic S L E) and follows prolonged ingestion of certain drugs (Table 12.4). All

Table 12.4 Drugs implicated in the induction of a lupus like syndrome. (From Harman J and Portonova, P (1982) *Clinics in Rheumatic diseases* **8**, 122.)

Cardiovascular	Procainamide
	Quinidine
	Beta-blockers
Anti-microbial	Isoniazid
	Griseofulvin
	Nitrofurantoin
Anti-convulsants	Phenytoin
	Ethosuximide
	Primidone
Antihypertensive	Hydralazine
	Methyldopa
	Reserpine
Antithyroid	Prophylthiovracil
Psychotropic	Chlorpromazine
	Lithium carbonate
Miscellaneous	D-Penicillamine
	Oral contraceptives
	Phenylbutazone

these drugs may result in A N A and L E cell formation (possibly due to anti-histone antibodies) but the S L E symptom complex is far more rare. The disease most commonly presents as arthralgias and rashes. Most S L E features may occur though it differs from idiopathic S L E in a number of respects:

— renal disease is rare
— D N A antibodies are usually absent
— older age group affected

— resolves on withdrawal of the offending drug (sometimes slowly)
— genetic factors may be involved (hydralazine lupus occurs in slow acetylators and is probably more frequent in HLA-DR4 individuals).

Discoid lupus

An intermittent, though frequently chronic, skin lesion which is occasionally associated with the systemic features of SLE.

CLINICAL FEATURES

Skin
— more clinically florid than the rash of SLE
— follicular plugging, scarring and scaling
— scarring alopecia
— mouth ulcers often chronic.

Other features
— older mean age group than SLE
— approximately 5% of patients develop systemic features, though these may be transitory
— ANA and LE cells occasionally seen
— chronic (RA-like) arthritis may occur.

INVESTIGATIONS IN SLE (*see* p. 21 for more details of laboratory investigations)

ANTINUCLEAR ANTIBODIES

ANA (usually in high titres, e.g. dilutions of 1 in 256 or more) are seen in the 95–99% of SLE patients.

'ANA negative-lupus' is rare—a small number of SLE patients with predominantly cutaneous features have persistently negative ANA. Some of these patients have anti-cytoplasmic (anti-Ro or anti-SSA) antibodies. In others, ANA appear after months or years of disease.

Anti-DNA antibodies. Antibodies against double stranded DNA provide the most specific diagnostic proof of SLE. These antibodies are found in 80–95% of patients with clinically active SLE, and are rarely found in other conditions.

Although the highest titres are generally found in patients with the most active disease, the correlation with disease activity in general is not close, some patients maintaining high titres of circulating anti-DNA antibodies for long periods despite little clinical evidence of disease activity.

LE CELLS

Though not specific, are found in 80% of SLE patients. Now superseded by fluorescent ANA (more sensitive) and DNA-binding tests (more specific).

COMPLEMENT

Lowered total haemolytic complement (CH_{50}) levels, as well as lowered levels of individual complement component levels (C3 and C4 levels most widely measured) are a sign of SLE disease activity. Although not a direct indication of renal disease, a rapidly falling CH_{50} suggests consumption by circulating immune complexes and *potential* renal damage.

IMMUNE COMPLEXES

Raised levels of circulating immune complexes by any of the 40-plus methods are detected in the serum of the majority of patients with active SLE, and are an important feature of the disease. Perhaps the simplest clinical test for complexes is the estimation of cryoprecipitates. (Fig. 12.5).

FALSE-POSITIVE TESTS FOR SYPHILIS

A positive WR or VDRL test, with a negative fluorescent treponema pallidum antibody test, is found in some 10% of SLE patients, often in association with a circulating anticoagulant. It is now known to be strongly associated with the tendency to thrombosis and to spontaneous abortion.

ESR AND C-REACTIVE PROTEIN

One of the striking features of SLE is the disparity between the acute phase responses. Even in active disease, high CRP levels are unusual, and it is not uncommon to see patients with ESR

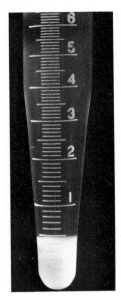

Fig. 12.5 Cryoprecipitate obtained after 72 hours at 4°C from a patient with SLE.

rates of at least 100 mm/hour and CRP values of near zero. A low CRP in a woman with active, suspected SLE is of great diagnostic value.

IMMUNOGLOBULINS

There is usually a polyclonal increase in gammaglobulins.

RADIOLOGY

Joint disease, where present, is usually non-erosive. Chest X-rays may show pleural thickening or effusions, atelectases, or (rarely) bilateral elevation of the diaphragms.

DIAGNOSIS AND DIFFERENTIAL DIAGNOSIS

The diagnosis of SLE in 'classical' form is straightforward. However, in many patients, the disease has been present for years before diagnosis. A number of useful clinical pointers in making a diagnosis in a patient with an unexplained multisystem disorder where S L E is suspected are given below:

Sex   Rare in the male

Age   Under 40

Race   Probably commoner in black females

Absence of erosions   in a patient with more than three years' arthritis

Leucopenia   Total W B C of over 7000 is unusual in S L E patients, but this may rise with infection and on institution of steroid therapy. Lymphopenia is often marked.

Other characteristic features.

— multiple drug allergies
— alopecia
— neuropsychiatric disturbances
— elbow vasculitis
— serology. The *absence* of anti D N A antibodies weighs very heavily against, but does not absolutely exclude a diagnosis of active S L E.

AMERICAN RHEUMATISM ASSOCIATION CRITERIA

In 1979 the A R A proposed classification criteria for S L E. This was revised in 1982 (Table 12.5).

Table 12.5   ARA revised criteria for classification of SLE.

Criteria

Malar rash
Discoid rash
Photosensitivity
Oral/nasal ulcers
Non-deforming arthritis (two or more joints)
Serositis (pleurisy or pericarditis)
Renal disease
CNS disease
Haematological disease (anaemia, leucopenia, lymphopenia or thrombocytopenia)
Immunological abnormalities (LE cells, anti-dsDNA, anti-Sm, positive VDRL/TPHA)
Antinuclear antibody (by immunofluorescence)

MANAGEMENT

MILD CASES

The majority of SLE patients can ultimately be weaned off all therapy. In patients with abnormal serological tests who are clinically well, current practice is to treat conservatively.

NON-STEROIDAL ANTI-INFLAMMATORY DRUGS

The first line drugs in patients with predominantly articular disease. Aspirin in full doses frequently causes hepatotoxicity in active SLE and is best avoided.

ANTIMALARIALS

Hydroxychloroquine 200 mg daily is particularly useful for patients with predominant skin and joint manifestations. Mepacrine is also useful but causes yellow pigmentation. Six-monthly eye checks are recommended, though the low doses now used give little danger of significant retinal toxicity.

CORTICOSTEROIDS

Prednisolone forms the cornerstone of management. It is given in high doses (60 mg daily) for severe disease (e.g. widespread vasculitis, acute nephritis, severe CNS vasculitis); or in moderate doses (10–30 mg daily) for less severe features (e.g. pleural effusions, moderate thrombocytopenia). Reduction of steroid doses to below 15 mg daily can often be achieved through an alternate day regime. Doses over 80 mg daily are rarely indicated.

IMMUNOSUPPRESSIVES

Azathioprine (2.5 mg/kg daily) plays a useful role as a steroid-sparing agent in SLE, especially in vasculitis. Cyclophosphamide is more toxic but useful in severe diffuse proliferative nephritis.

'PULSE' THERAPY

Intermittent boluses of drugs given intravenously are currently being tried in a number of centres, e.g. methylprednisolone 1 g on 3 successive days (repeated 3–4 weekly if necessary) and cyclophosphamide 500 mg i.v. stat and 150 mg weekly. It is hoped that intravenous therapy will have a more immediate and profound immunosuppressive effect, but this form of therapy is still experimental.

PLASMA EXCHANGE (PLASMAPHERESIS)

This involves the intermittent removal of 2–4 l blood which is then centrifuged; the cells are returned to the patient together with a plasma substitute. The procedure presumably removes, amongst other things, immune complexes, fibrin products, and complement components. Although of great theoretical interest in SLE, plasma exchange has not yet been adequately assessed.

PROGNOSIS

The 10 year survival from SLE is now well in the 90% range, largely due to the recognition of milder forms of the disease. Deaths still occur from severe vasculitis and renal disease, but it is hoped that deaths from infection in heavily immunosuppressed and cushingoid patients will become relatively less common as more moderation with these drugs becomes practice. Although the classical pattern is one of exacerbation and remission, it is not uncommon to see a pattern characterised by a severe initial flare followed by prolonged mild or negligible disease activity.

13　Scleroderma

Scleroderma is a chronic disease characterised by widespread sclerosis of collagen, predominently affecting skin, but also affecting the gastrointestinal tract, heart, muscles and lungs. Because of the widespread visceral involvement, the alternative name 'systemic sclerosis' is preferred by many. A number of forms of scleroderma are recognised:
— progressive systemic sclerosis
— scleroderma of the skin (morphoea, localised or diffuse)
— CREST
— mixed connective tissue disease.
These variants, although discussed separately, contain many similarities and considerable overlap exists.

EPIDEMIOLOGY

Prevalence　Scleroderma is a rare disease with an incidence of approximately 3 per million population.

Sex　The female:male ratio is 9:1.

Age at onset　Any age; commonest at 30–50 years.

Geography　Possibly commonest in some black races though this is uncertain. Commoner in some mining communities.

AETIOLOGY

The aetiology of scleroderma is unknown. Contributing factors include:

EXCESSIVE SYNTHESIS OF COLLAGEN

The stimulus to this synthesis is unknown. Silica has been implicated in some of the mining groups as well as in a rare scleroderma-like disease following silicon breast implants (graft *vs* host disease).

MICROVASCULAR LESIONS

A widespread micro-angiopathy (as demonstrated by nailfold capillaroscopy) is thought by some to antedate the collagen changes.

IMMUNOLOGICAL

In early scleroderma, immunological changes include antinuclear antibodies, hypergammaglobulinaemia and circulating complexes. In some cases, sensitised lymphocytes have been shown to stimulate fibroblast and endothelial cell proliferation.

GENETIC

An increased prevalence of H L A-D R5 has been shown in some studies.

PATHOLOGY

SKIN

Early changes include oedema and perivascular lymphocytic infiltrates.
Later there is an increase in dermal collagen, a reduction in elastic tissue, and a chronic vasculitis of small blood vessels.
Late changes include scarring and loss of secondary appendages such as sweat glands.

OTHER ORGANS

The pathology is similar in most organs and includes fibrosis, widespread increase in collagen, sclerosis of blood vessels, and secondary atrophy (e.g. of muscle)
Particular organ features are:
Gastrointestinal tract
Rigidity and loss of motility, secondary oesophagitis and ulceration, small bowel superinfection ('stagnant loop').
Lung
Pulmonary fibrosis; especially lower lobes; pulmonary capillary basement membrane thickening; pulmonary hypertension.
Muscle
Myopathy and/or myositis.

Heart
Pericarditis; cardiomyopathy; conduction tissue fibrosis.

Kidney
Fibrinoid in arteriole walls; changes resembling malignant hypertension.

CLINICAL FEATURES

The disease may present dramatically, with visible, rapid progression over a period of weeks or, more commonly, it may present in a gradual, insidious way.

Raynaud's phenomenon

This is the commonest feature and is generally early and severe. It may precede other features by many years. Conversely, scleroderma should be considered high on the list of causes of Raynaud's developing after the age of 30.

Skin

In addition to the features of Raynaud's, early changes include hyperpigmentation (or occasionally vitiligo in pigmented skin), thickening and tightening. This is clinically best appreciated in the fingers, around the eyelids (especially in the normally lax lower eyelid) and around the mouth and nose. Late changes include dermal atrophy, ulceration, calcification, and telangiectases.

Gastrointestinal tract

MOUTH

Sicca syndrome.
Thickening of peridontal membrane (leads to characteristic dental X-ray appearances).
Small mouth aperture.
Telangiectases of lips.

OESOPHAGUS (Fig. 13.1)

Abnormal oesophageal hypomotility probably occurs in the majority of cases.

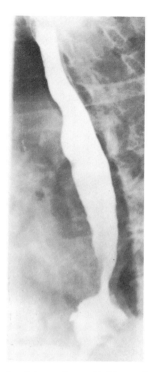

Fig. 13.1 Absent peristalsis and small hiatus hernia in scleroderma. These appearances in themselves are not pathonognomic, and screening or manometry is required to demonstrate the uncoordinated contractions.

Reflux oesophagitis and oesophageal ulceration.
Ultimately oesophageal stricture may result.
Note   A 'normal' barium swallow does not exclude oesophageal dysfunction.

LIVER, STOMACH AND DUODENUM

Fibrosis and atrophy in stomach and duodenum.
Duodenal atrophy and dilation.

SMALL BOWEL

Malabsorption syndrome (scleroderma involvement $\pm$ stagnant loop syndrome).

Dilatation (especially proximal jejunum).
Jejunal sacculation.

COLON

Dilatation of the whole of the large bowel may be prominent.
Wide-mouthed diverticulae, when present, are particularly suggestive of scleroderma.
Pneumatosis cystoides intestinalis (rare).

Liver

An association between primary biliary cirrhosis and scleroderma and its variants (especially the CRST syndrome) is well described (*see below*).

Lung

Lung involvement probably occurs in the majority of patients with systemic sclerosis, though widespread pulmonary fibrosis is seen in less than 50%.
Other pulmonary features include:
— reflux pneumonitis: a late manifestation
— chest infections: a common cause of death in severe systemic sclerosis
— pulmonary hypertension: often insidious, presenting clinically at a late stage
— bronchiolar carcinoma: a rare complication of chronic pulmonary fibrosis
— pleural thickening and calcification
— pulmonary vasculitis: rare.
Clinical and investigative findings include: dyspnoea, medium or coarse crepitations, basal mottling and linear densities on X-ray, (Fig. 13.2) and restrictive ventilatory impairment and reduced transfer factor.

Cardiovascular system

Myocarditis: ECG abnormalities common and often subtle.
Pericarditis: may occur at any stage of the disease.
Conduction tissue fibrosis: arrhythmias and sudden death.

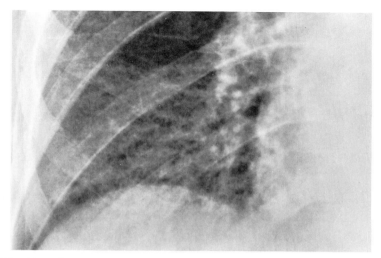

Fig. 13.2 Lung detail in a patient with diffuse systemic sclerosis (scleroderma). Diffuse interstitial fibrosis in the lung causes a reticular pattern which is always best seen in the bases. (Dr David Lewall, King Faisal Specialist Hospital, Saudi Arabia.)

Kidney

Usually a late manifestation. Hypertension is prominent and a grave prognostic sign. Both hypertensive and renal failure may be rapidly progressive.

Muscles

Myopathy is common and sometimes early (earlier figures may have underemphasised its incidence). Myositis with raised muscle enzymes is occasionally seen.

Tendons and joints

Tendon crepitation and stiffness are common, while joint stiffness and limitation result from rigid periarticular tissues; inflammatory arthritis is uncommon.

LABORATORY INVESTIGATIONS

ESR

A useful sign of disease activity, but often normal in late and end-stage disease.

C-reactive protein
As in SLE, the CRP may remain normal in the face of a raised ESR.

Antinuclear antibodies
Positive in up to 60% of early cases. 'Speckled' or 'nucleolar' patterns are common (*see* p. 22).

Blood: Anaemia
Normochromic, normocytic (commonest).
Macrocytic (malabsorption).
Haemolytic (rare), often transient.
Iron deficiency, often associated with hiatus hernia.

Special investigations
Skin biopsy may be helpful in early diagnosis.
EMG and muscle enzymes for myositis.
B_{12} and folate; faecal fat estimation for malabsorption.
ECG: conduction defects; myocarditis.
Pulmonary function tests.
Renal function tests.

RADIOLOGY

X-ray changes may include:
— hands: loss of tufts of terminal phalanges; soft tissue calcification
— chest: basal fibrosis, pulmonary hypertension
— gastrointestinal tract: oesophageal dilation and poor motility, widened and 'rigid' duodenal loop
— abnormal small bowel
— wide-mouthed diverticulae of large bowel.

MANAGEMENT

RAYNAUD'S PHENOMENON

The most important and useful measures include:
— no smoking

— avoidance of cold; both to the extremities and body generally
— avoidance of drugs which cause peripheral vasoconstriction, e.g. ergotamine containing agents, beta-blockers
— strict care of finger pulp ulceration and infection
— nifedipine is an effective oral agent in some patients
— intra-arterial reserpine may be useful when Raynaud's causes severe and prolonged digital ischaemia but it should be administered by an expert in arterial injection
— other agents include various vasodilators, antifibrinolytic and antiplatelet drugs, the role and efficacy of which remain uncertain
— surgical sympathectomy is rarely indicated since its beneficial effect is typically transient.

SCLERODERMA (skin involvement)

The following drugs may be employed:
— D-penicillamine may be beneficial in early cases
— colchicine remains under evaluation
— corticosteroids are only indicated in some cases of progressive and rapid skin involvement where oedema is the dominant feature.

VISCERAL INVOLVEMENT

There is no specific drug treatment for systemic involvement. Important symptomatic measures include:
— prompt treatment of reflux oesophagitis, including the use of H2 antagonists when necessary
— dilatation of oesophageal strictures
— broad spectrum antibiotics for 'stagnant-loop' syndrome
— rapid and effective control of hypertension and renal failure
— corticosteroids for haemolytic anaemia, acute pericarditis and inflammatory myositis.

PROGNOSIS

The five year survival rate is 75%.
The prognosis is related inversely to the degree of visceral involvement. In the individual patient, accurate prognosis is difficult. An apparently rapidly progressive disease may become quiescent.

VARIANTS OF SCLERODERMA

Mixed connective tissue disease (MCTD)

This condition was originally defined serologically, with the presence of antibodies against ribonucleo-protein (RNP). It was found that individuals whose sera contained anti-RNP antibodies (and no other antibodies) showed certain clinical similarities, with 'overlap' features of scleroderma, systemic lupus, and myositis. Although it was initially felt that MCTD was a distinct syndrome, time has shown that many patients in this group changed the pattern of their disease (and their antibodies), notably to more 'classical' scleroderma.

SEROLOGICAL FEATURES

Antibodies against RNP
— usually in high titre
— absence of other autoantibodies (including anti-DNA antibodies)
Hyperglobulinaemia
— speckled pattern ANA

CLINICAL FEATURES

Raynaud's
— severe, prominent, early.
— a major cause of morbidity.
Arthritis
— often prominent.— 'sausage fingers' from synovitis
— tendonitis and skin oedema.
Myositis
— usually mild.
Features of SLE
— cerebritis, rashes, serositis and vasculitis.
— renal disease is rare.
Features of scleroderma
— some patients with MCTD gradually progress to chronic systemic sclerosis.

PROGNOSIS

Initially this was thought to be good, as renal disease is rare. However, morbidity, especially from Raynaud's, is often severe.

Other 'overlap' syndromes

An increasing number of autoantibodies are now recognised. In parallel with these discoveries, attempts have been made to associate various members of the spectrum of lupus-scleroderma–myositis with these antibodies. Some of the currently described associations are listed in Table 13.1.

Table 13.1 Autoantibodies associated with S L E—scleroderma-myositis spectrum

Disease	Antibody against
Seronegative lupus ⎱ I T P ⎰ Ro (S S A) Sjögren's ⎰	Ro (S S A)
Sjögren's	La (S S B)
M C T D	R N P
Polymyositis and pulmonary fibrosis	Jo-1
C R E S T	Centromere
Scleroderma	Scl 70

Cutaneous scleroderma

Cutaneous scleroderma (morphoea) may be local or widespread. In localised scleroderma many variants are recognised, e.g. linear, 'coup de sabre' (an elongated scar, often down the forehead and face), or hemiatrophy. Note that underlying muscle wasting and fibrosis may be considerable. These patients rarely develop systemic features.

C R E S T (Calcinosis, Raynaud's oesophagitis,) Sclerodactyly, Telangiectasia)

Although many patients with the C R E S T syndrome have, or later develop, signs of systemic sclerosis, this variant of scleroderma is usually clinically distinctive:
— calcinosis may affect finger tips Fig. 13.3, subcutaneous tissue on elbows and knees and may ulcerate
— telangiectases are widespread; they mimic hereditary telangiectasia, but rarely bleed

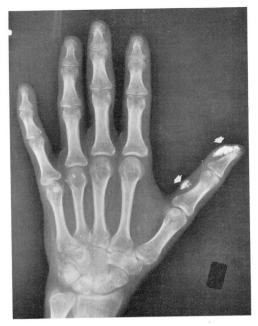

Fig. 13.3 CREST syndrome. This is a variant of diffuse systemic sclerosis (scleroderma) with less servere visceral involvment. There is calcinosis (arrows). (Dr David Lewall, King Faisal Specialist Hospital, Saudi Arabia.)

— pulmonary hypertension is now recognised as a late complication
— some cases are associated with primary biliary cirrhosis
— serologically the patient may have anti-centromere antibodies.

Eosinophilic fasciitis

Although not obviously related to scleroderma, this condition may mimic acute scleroderma.

FEATURES

Diffuse fasciitis (subcutaneous and not cutaneous). The affected area (often forearm or calf) feels tense and woody. There is blood eosinophilia (and sometimes tissue eosinophilia) but no systemic involvement.

AETIOLOGY

Unknown, but said to follow unusually hard muscular work in some cases.

PROGNOSIS

Good, though late marrow failure and late development of localised scleroderma have been reported.

14 Dermatomyositis and Polymyositis

This is an inflammatory disease of muscle, with an associated skin rash in 25% of patients.

CLASSIFICATION

1 Childhood polymyositis: vasculitis is prominent; considered by many to be distinct from adult polymyositis.
2 Idiopathic dermatomyositis.
3 Myositis associated with a connective tissue disorder (e.g. Sjögren's syndrome, scleroderma, SLE).
4 Myositis associated with malignancy.

EPIDEMIOLOGY

Prevalence Unknown.

Sex The female:male ratio is 3:2.

Age All age groups. Adult disease commoner in 40 to 60 year-olds.

AETIOLOGY

Host T lymphocytes are directly involved in muscle cell killing. The factor (or factors) activating these lymphocytes is unknown.

INFECTIVE

Paramyxovirus-like particles seen in some muscle biopsies; raised antibody titres to Coxsackie B group viruses seen in some cases.

ASSOCIATION WITH OTHER CONNECTIVE TISSUE DISEASES

In common with other connective tissue diseases, e.g. Sjögren's syndrome, an association with H L A-B8 has been found.

ASSOCIATION WITH MALIGNANCY

The strength of the association with malignancy is unknown, though recent evidence suggests that it is uncommon. A 'blind' search for malignancy is almost certainly unwarranted. Childhood dermatomyositis is not associated with malignancy.

PATHOLOGY

MUSCLE

Inflammatory muscle infiltrate—mainly lymphocytes.
Necrosis of muscle fibres with patchy regeneration.
Later, fibrosis, atrophy.

SKIN

Collagenous thickening of the dermis.
Dermal infiltration with chronic inflammatory cells (often perivascular).

CLINICAL FEATURES

MUSCLE

Acute
The hallmark of the disease is weakness (e.g. rising from a chair, climbing stairs)
— symmetrical
— proximal weakness is usually more prominent
— respiratory muscle weakness is usually late
— tenderness of muscle is surprisingly uncommon.

Chronic
The features of chronic disease are atrophy, contractures (occasionally severe in children), and calcinosis (occasionally widespread) Fig. 14.1.

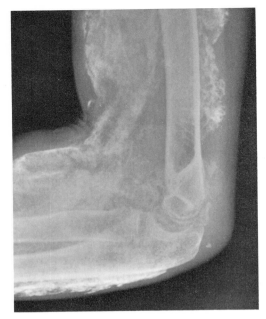

Fig. 14.1   Dermatomyositis in an 11 year old girl. The calcification is in muscles and other soft tissues deep to the subcutaneous layers. (Dr David Lewall, King Faisal Specialist Hospital, Saudi Arabia.)

Note:
Muscle strength is as good a guide to disease activity as enzymes or any other measurement.

SKIN

Acute
— characteristic 'heliotrope', purple rash on eyelids and light-exposed areas often with oedema
— scaly 'collodion' patches on the knuckles (Gottron's patches) and extensor surfaces
— skin ulceration
— periungual capillary dilation, especially prominent in children
— oedema over acutely inflamed muscle groups
— Raynaud's phenomenon
— thickening of finger skin, sometimes resembling scleroderma
— telangiectasia

SYSTEMIC FEATURES

The muscle weakness may pass unnoticed in the patient with a 'systemic' onset with fever, weight loss, arthralgias, arthritis (usually transient), splenomegaly and Raynaud's phenomenon.

GASTROINTESTINAL TRACT

Dysphagia (and pseudo-bulbar palsy with dysphonia).
Impaired oesophageal motility.
Rare oesophageal diverticulae.
Malignancy.

HEART AND BLOOD VESSELS

Cardiomyopathy: true incidence unknown.
Raynaud's phenomenon in up to 30%.
Rarely, adult myositis also associated with widespread vasculitis.

LUNGS

Respiratory muscle weakness and failure.
Aspiration pneumonitis.
Pulmonary infiltration: either acute (responds to steroids) or chronic fibrosing alveolitis.

DIAGNOSIS

NON-SPECIFIC

E S R raised in the acute state.
Antinuclear antibodies against a number of extractable nuclear components have been reported. Anti Jo-1 is notably associated with the tendency to pulmonary fibrosis.
Polyclonal hyperglobulinaemia.

MUSCLE ENZYMES

CPK, aldolase, SGOT: One or two, or all three enzymes are raised in most patients which is useful in monitoring adult disease activity but less valuable in children.

MUSCLE BIOPSY

Lesions are 'patchy' and, even in involved muscle, only 75% of biopsies show inflammation.
Biopsy may not be indicated in children.

ELECTROMYOGRAPHY

Typical features of myositis include:
— fibrillation
— polyphasic action potentials
— pseudomyotonic discharges.

MANAGEMENT

Prednisone up to 60 mg daily is used in acute severe cases, but the dose should be reduced as soon as a clinical response is obtained.
Methotrexate, azathioprine, or cyclophosphamide may be given in 'resistant' (i.e. unresponsive to prednisone after 8 weeks) cases.
Removal of associated neoplasm produces a variable response in myositis.
Experimental forms of therapy in severe cases include total body irradiation, thoracic duct drainage and plasmapheresis.

PROGNOSIS

The cumulative survival rate is 70% at two years, followed by a levelling; this suggests that early effective treatment might result in improved overall prognosis. In uncomplicated ANA-negative idiopathic polymyositis recurrence after early effective treatment is unusual.

15 Sjögren's Syndrome

Two forms of Sjögren's syndrome are recognised: the complete form and the limited or primary form.

COMPLETE FORM

The complete form consists of:
— sicca complex: keratoconjunctivitis sicca (dry eyes) and xerostomia (dry mouth)
and
— a connective tissue disorder: usually rheumatoid arthritis.

LIMITED OR PRIMARY FORM

The limited or primary form (also called the sicca syndrome) consists of:
— sicca complex
with or *without*
— variable systemic manifestations.

EPIDEMIOLOGY

Prevalence   Occurs in 10–30% of patients with rheumatoid arthritis.

Sex   Predominantly female (80–90%).

Age   Usually middle-aged but any age can be affected.

AETIOLOGY

Unknown but considered to be an 'autoimmune' disease to which patients are genetically predisposed.

PATHOLOGY

The essential lesion consists of
1   chronic lymphocytic infiltrate of:
Salivary glands:
— major: parotid submaxillary
— minor: gingival, palatine.
— lacrimal glands.
Other exocrine glands in the:
— respiratory tract
— gastrointestinal tract
— skin and vagina.
The infiltrate can cause glandular enlargement.
2   Acinar atrophy and proliferative changes in the duct lining
cells also takes place.

Diminished secretions from the affected glands are responsible
for the manifestations of the sicca syndrome.

CLINICAL MANIFESTATIONS

Ocular (Keratoconjunctivitis sicca)

Persistent grittiness or foreign body sensations.
Accumulation of ropy mucus Fig. 15.1.

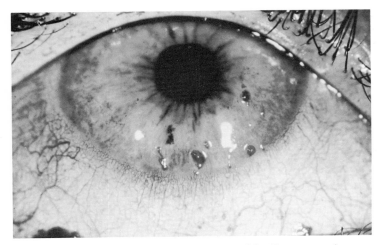

Fig. 15.1 Corneal vascularisation and keratitis filamentosa in severe
Sjögren's syndrome. (Mr Peter Wright, Moorfields Hospital, London.)

Photosensitivity or tiredness of the eyes.
Inability to produce tears in response to emotional or chemical stimulants.
Eye examination usually normal but mild conjunctivitis or mucus accumulation may be evident.
Lacrimal gland enlargement is rare.
The first symptoms of involvement may be excessive mucus accumulation rather than complaints of dry eyes.
Lack of tear secretion predisposes to infection.

Oral (Xerostomia)

Difficulty chewing, swallowing and phonating.
Fissures and ulcers of the tongue or mucous membranes.
Dental caries.
Firm, generally non-tender parotid gland enlargement in some patients and submaxillary gland enlargement in a few.

Other Features of Sicca Syndrome

Nasal dryness and epistaxes.
Otitis media.
Hoarseness.
Bronchitis, pneumonia, pleurisy.
Dry skin.
Vaginitis sicca.

Accompanying Diseases

Diseases occurring with the sicca syndrome to constitute the complete form of Sjögren's syndrome include:
Rheumatoid arthritis:
— invariably seropositive
— this is the connective tissue disorder in about 90% of patients with the complete form.
Systemic lupus erythematosus.
Progressive systemic sclerosis.
Polymyositis.
Rarely:
— vasculitis
— Hashimoto's thyroiditis

— biliary cirrhosis
— active chronic hepatitis.

Other Associations

Other associations of the complete or limited forms of Sjögren's syndrome include:
Raynaud's phenomenon.
Splenomegaly.
Hepatomegaly.
Lymphadenopathy.
Hyperglobulinaemic purpura.
Renal tubular abnormalities.
Pulmonary fibrosis.
Peripheral neuropathy and proximal myopathy.
Increased incidence of allergic reactions to drugs. This has clear implications with regard to the drug treatment. of associated diseases such as R A.

LABORATORY FINDINGS

Anaemia: usually normochromic, normocytic.
Leukopenia and eosinophilia may be found.
E S R is raised, often to very high levels.
Hypergammaglobulinaemia; cryoglobulinaemia sometimes found.
Rheumatoid factor—positive in 80–100%. IgA RF may predominate.
Antinuclear antibodies—positive in 60–80%
— antibodies to a range of non-histone antigens or extractable nuclear antigens including Ro, La, and others produce a typically speckled pattern of immunofluorescence
— L E cell test is positive in 10–20%.
Other autoantibodies are common:
— Sjögren's syndrome is second only to S L E in the range of autoantibodies which are found. These include antibodies to:
    thyroglobulin
    smooth muscle
    gastric parietal cells
    salivary duct epithelium
— the last occurs in up to 50% of patients but is not specific and therefore lacks diagnostic value.

HLA associations:
- primary Sjögren's syndrome is associated with increased frequency of HLA-B8 and DR3
- Sjögren's syndrome with rheumatoid arthritis is associated with HLA-DR4.

The discrepancy between HLA-DR3 and DR4 in these groups suggests that genetic predisposition is different in the two forms of Sjögren's syndrome.

DIAGNOSIS

The diagnosis of the sicca syndrome can be strongly suspected on clinical grounds but objective evidence of lacrimal and salivary glandular abnormality can be obtained by the following special investigations.

To confirm keratoconjunctivitis sicca

SCHIRMER'S TEST (Fig. 15.2)

The length of wetting of a standardised strip of filter paper, inserted into the conjunctival sac (hooked over the lower eyelid) for 5 minutes as shown in the figure, gives some indication of eye dryness. Wetting of over 15 mm is normal; less than 5 mm

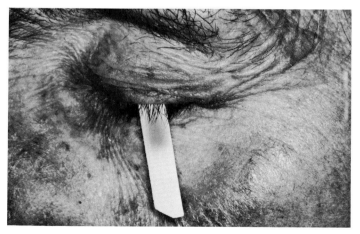

Fig. 15.2 Schirmer's test. Wetting of less than 15 mm of the test paper in 5 minutes is regarded as abnormal.

abnormal and 5-15 mm, equivocal. This simple, rapid test is of value in screening patients for Sjögren's syndrome if performed under the conditions specified by the makers of Schirmer's papers, which are available from any eye department.

ROSE BENGAL TEST

A solution of Rose Bengal (1%) is instilled into the conjunctival sac and washed out with sterile saline. Conjunctival abrasions due to keratoconjunctivitis sicca are stained with the dye.

SLIT LAMP EXAMINATION

This is the definitive examination for keratoconjunctivitis sicca and may show:
— increased corneal debris
— attached filaments of corneal epithelium (filamentary keratitis)
— punctate keratitis.

To confirm salivary gland abnormality

Parotid salivary flow rate: diminished.
Secretory sialography: shows distortion of the normal pattern of parotid ductules.

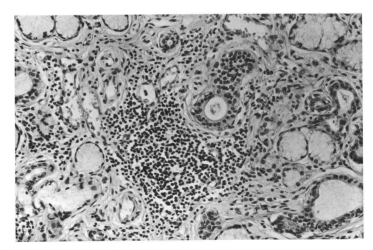

Fig. 15.3 Labial salivary gland biopsy showing a periductal focus of lymphocytes together with moderate diffuse lymphocytic infiltration (× 210). (Dr D Chisholm, Dundee University Dental Hospital.)

Salivary scintigraphy demonstrates diminished uptake of technetium pertechnetate on scanning.
Biopsy of minor salivary glands of the lip will confirm lymphocytic infiltrate (Fig. 15.3).
Of most practical value are the full eye assessment and in cases of diagnostic difficulty, biopsy of a minor salivary gland.

DIFFERENTIAL DIAGNOSIS

Salivary gland enlargement may be caused by:
Sjögren's syndrome.
Sarcoidosis.
Lymphoma.
Waldenström's macroglobulinaemia.
Cirrhosis of the liver.
Xerostomia may be due to:
Sjögren's syndrome.
Drugs, e.g. tricyclic antidepressants.
Mouth breathing.

COMPLICATIONS

With ketatoconjunctivitis sicca there may be infection and/or corneal damage.
With glandular and extraglandular lymphocytic infiltration there may be pseudolymphoma and/or lymphoma.
Although lymphoma is uncommon it should be considered in patients with prominent lymph node enlargement or salivary gland enlargement, infiltrates of kidneys or lungs and falling immunoglobulin levels.

COURSE

Usually protracted but mild.
In patients severely affected by Sjögren's syndrome, extreme discomfort and suffering can be caused by the sicca components.
It does not influence the course of rheumatoid arthritis.

MANAGEMENT

There is no treatment available at present which will cure Sjögren's syndrome. Steroids are of limited value. Immunosuppressives such as cyclophosphamide may improve lacrimal and salivary secretions but such potentially toxic treatment is rarely indicated. The presence of Sjögren's syndrome does not affect the management of rheumatoid arthritis except insofar as these patients are more liable to show allergic reactions to drugs.

Keratoconjunctivitis sicca:

— artificial tears, in the form of methylcellulose drops should be instilled into the conjunctival sac as often as necessary to keep the eyes moist
— in patients with some residual tear formation, nasolacrimal duct occlusion may be helpful.

Xerostoma:

— difficult to treat
— frequent sips of fluid provides some relief
— control local infection, e.g. Candida.

16 Vasculitis

Vasculitis is the inflammation of blood vessels. In clinical practice the term covers a variety of histological types, from a predominantly polymorph infiltration to granulomatous inflammation, as well as a broad spectrum of vessel involvement. The classification of vasculitis remains unsatisfactory. Pathological criteria are based on vessel size, intensity of inflammatory response, and degree of granuloma formation. For clinical purposes, the following simple division into primary and secondary vasculitis is proposed.

Primary

Polyarteritis nodosa.
Granulomatous arteritis (including Wegener's granuloma).
Allergic and cutaneous vasculitis (including serum sickness and Henoch–Schoenlein purpura).
Takayasu's arteritis.
Giant cell arteritis.

Secondary (associated with other systemic disease features)

S L E.
Rheumatoid arthritis.
Scleroderma.
Childhood dermatomyositis.
Associated with malignancy, infection and drugs.

POLYARTERITIS NODOSA

This is an intense inflammatory condition of small and medium sized arteries. The infiltrate is largely polymorphonuclear cells. The lesions are frequently segmental and occur at junctions of vessels. The distribution of lesions leads to widespread and severe clinical features.

Epidemiology

Incidence   Classical polyarteritis nodosa is one of the rarest of the connective tissue diseases.

Sex   The male:female ratio is 4:1 (the only major connective tissue disease with a male predominance).

Age   All age groups affected.

Aetiology

Associated with hepatitis B infection in 10–20% of patients. Almost certainly related to hepatitis B surface antigen-containing immune complexes in these patients.

Hypersensitivity (occasional cases follow sulphonamides or penicillin).

Increased incidence in heroin and other drug addiction (?associated with hepatitis infection in some).

A PAN-like condition has been seen in a small number of cases of hairy cell leukaemia (antigen unknown).

Pathology

MICROSCOPIC

PAN is the most inflammatory of the arteritides, with intense polymorph infiltration of all layers of medium sized arteries, leading to degeneration (including fibrinoid change), weakness, and aneurysm formation. Veins and vasa nervorum may be affected. Vascular inflammation and thrombosis lead to tissue infarction.

MACROSCOPIC CHANGES

Infarction may occur in any organ.

Clinical features

GENERAL

PAN is usually a severe and dramatic illness. It frequently starts with calf pain and with general malaise, myalgias, weight loss, and joint pains. This prodromal phase may last days before more clear-cut visceral manifestations occur.

CIRCULATORY

— livedo reticularis
— digital gangrene
— intermittent claudication
— thrombophlebitis (occasionally thrombophlebitis migrans).

HEART

Changes may include:
— tachycardia (may indicate myocarditis)
— arrhythmias
— vasculitis of the coronary vessels may lead to death from cardiac infarction
— pericarditis
— hypertensive changes.

SKIN

A variety of skin rashes occur, notably livedo reticularis. Purpura is unusual in classical PAN.

KIDNEY

An acute immune-complex glomerulitis may occur. Much more important, however, are vascular changes in the kidney. The two commonest clinical features are haematuria (often microscopic) and hypertension.

GASTROINTESTINAL

Up to two-thirds of patients present with abdominal pain. The main clinical presentations are:
— 'acute abdomen' (infarction of viscera; peritonitis)
— malabsorbtion syndrome (rare)
— liver tenderness (gall bladder and liver infarction occasionally occur).

NERVOUS SYSTEM

Although mononeuritis multiplex is the best well known manifestation of PAN, a wide spectrum of neurological abnormalities

may be seen either in the central nervous system:
— psychosis or confusion
— retinopathy
— hemiparesis
— cranial nerval lesions
— brain stem lesions
or in the peripheral nervous system:
— mononeuritis multiplex—60%
— mixed mono and polyneuritis
— polyneuritis.

EYE

The commonest changes in the fundus are those of hypertension: exudates in the absence of·hypertension ('cytoid bodies') result from leakage from inflamed ocular vessels. The main ocular manifestations of PAN are:
— haemorrhages, exudates, papilloedema
— uveitis, iritis, keratitis, scleritis, conjunctivitis
— field defects
— primary optic atrophy
— corneal ulceration.

LUNGS

Lungs are not typically involved in classical PAN; the subgroup of patients with eosinophilia and lung involvement have been separated into the entity known as the Churg–Strauss syndrome. In 20% of cases asthma is an early manifestation. Some 95% of these cases have eosinophilia and pulmonary infiltrates may be seen on chest X-ray.

EAR, NOSE AND THROAT

Although ENT involvement is well recognised in Wegner's granulomatosis, it is common for both classical as well as atypical PAN to present with rhinitis, otitis, or hearing difficulties. A subset of patients with arteritis following serous otitis externa has been described.

Polyarteritis in children

Children as young as 2-3 years may develop PAN.
Clinical features include the following:
— transient macular exanthem
— transient conjunctivitis
— pyrexia
— congestive failure
— frequent ECG changes.
Familial cases have been recorded. Aneurysms of the coronary tree have been a prominent finding at autopsy. A severe exanthematous eruption with lymphadenopathy and coronary vasculitis (Kawasaki's syndrome) is becoming recognised in children not only in Japan, where large numbers of infants have been diagnosed, but elsewhere. The cause is unknown.

Investigations

GENERAL

The most useful general guides to disease activity are the neutrophil count (less commonly the eosinophil count), the ESR, and urine microscopy. It is not unusual to see polymorph counts of 20 000–30 000 mm³ in severe cases.

ANGIOGRAPHY (Fig. 16.1)

The most important investigation and, in good hands, more useful than 'blind' muscle biopsy. Multiple aneurysms of the renal vessels or coeliac axis branches are seen in up to 80% of active PAN cases.

MUSCLE BIOPSY

The 'positive yield' varies between 13 and 50%. Only clinically involved muscle should be biopsied and 'blind' muscle biopsy is probably unwarranted.

Management

Corticosteroids: the dose is based largely on clinical criteria, but initial doses of 60 mg prednisolone daily are usually required.

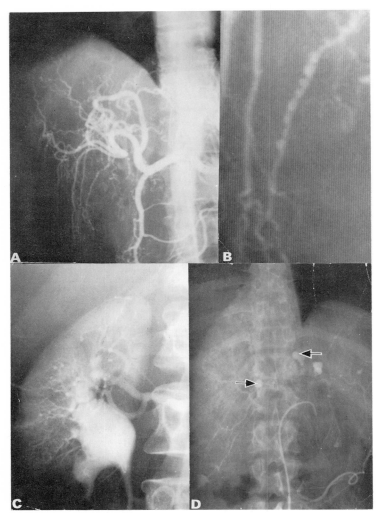

Fig. 16.1   Arteriography in polyarteritis nodosa. Selective coeliac axis angiogram showing small aneurysms in the hepatic arteries, **A**. The multiple nature of the changes is well seen on a magnification study, **B**. In many patients, the aneurysms are most readily demonstrated in the renal vascular bed, **C**. Late films in such renal series commonly show nephrographic defects due to multiple infarcts. The aneurysms depicted in A, B and C are fairly typical in size; however, occasionally larger lesions may be seen, **D**. (Professor David Allison, Royal Postgraduate Medical School, Hammersmith Hospital, London.)

Immunosuppressives: cyclophosphamide or another immunosuppressive is indicated in severe acute cases in addition to steroids. Strict and early management of hypertension and renal failure is required.

'Pulse' methylprednisolone and 'pulse' i.v. cyclophosphamide are being increasingly used in the early, active phase.

Prognosis

The 5-year survival rate is 50–60%.

Prognosis improves markedly after the first 3 months of disease and the majority of patients who survive classical 'PAN' do *not* have subsequent attacks of the disease after the first year.

WEGENER'S GRANULOMATOSIS

A rare form of necrotising vasculitis of the upper and lower respiratory tract associated with granuloma formation and nephritis.

Epidemiology

Incidence Rare.

Sex The ratio of males:females is 2:1.

Age Commoner after the age of 40.

Pathology

An inflammatory panarteritis—often slightly less intense than PAN, with a predominantly mononuclear infiltrate.

Necrotising granulomata of the respiratory tract.

Focal or diffuse proliferative nephritis.

Clinical features

RESPIRATORY TRACT

Upper respiratory tract features are prominent:
— sinusitis, rhinorrhoea
— ulceration of the nasal mucosa and cartilage.

LUNGS

Lung involvement is invariable:
— nodules, infiltrates, cavitation (Fig. 16.2), pleural effusions
— may be rapidly progressive
— chest infections complicate the clinical picture.

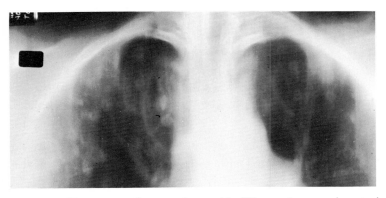

Fig. 16.2 Tomogram from patient with Wegener's granulomatosis showing multiple cavitating lesions. (Professor David Allison, Royal Postgraduate Medical School, Hammersmith Hospital, London.)

KIDNEY

Nephritis in 85%:
— rapidly progressive if untreated
— hypertension unusual (*see* PAN).

EYE

Changes may include:
— proptosis due to 'pseudotumour' of retro-orbital granulomatous tissue
— keratitis, conjunctivitis, uveitis
— direct extension of granulomatous tissue into brain.

Laboratory investigations

Normochronic, normocytic anaemia.
Neutrophilia and thrombocytosis.
Weakly positive rheumatoid factor in about 50% of patients.

Management and prognosis

Steroids: prednisolone in high doses (e.g. 60 mg/day) initially. Immunosuppressives: cyclophosphamide appears superior to azathioprine in this condition. 'Pulse' cyclophosphide useful in the early, acute stages. One of the striking features of Wegener's granulomatosis is that progression of disease and relapses both occur on steroids alone. Immunosuppressive therapy is mandatory.

Prognosis

The prognosis, once uniformly fatal within 1–2 years, has been dramatically improved by the advent of cyclophosphamide, though some long-term relapses are being reported.

CHURG-STRAUSS SYNDROME

Regarded by some as a variant of PAN or Wegener's granulomatosis, in 'classical' form this has enough distinguishing features to be regarded as a distinct syndrome.

Clinical features

Asthma ($\pm$ atopy). It is common for asthma to precede the vasculitis by up to 20 years.
Pulmonary infiltrates.
Systemic vasculitis.
Eosinophilia.
Pericarditis.
Myocarditis: one of the features which distinguishes Churg-Strauss syndrome from other vasculides is the high (up to 50%) incidence of cardiac and pericardial involvement.

'Limited' forms of the disease include eosinophilic pneumonia (Loeffler's syndrome) and localised or diffuse eosinophilic infiltration of the gastrointestinal tract.

TAKAYASU'S ARTERITIS

This is a chronic inflammatory arteritis of the aorta and its main branches. It typically affects young women between the ages of

20 and 30 and the largest number of cases have been reported from the Far East.

Clinical features

After an initial prodromal illness with weight loss, myalgia and synovitis, the 'vascular' phase begins with loss of pulses, typically affecting the upper limbs ('pulseless disease'). Involvement of other aortic branches may cause CVAs, ocular problems, coronary thrombosis, or hypertension (renal arteries). (Fig. 16.3.)

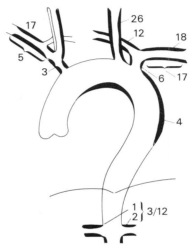

Fig. 16.3 Frequency of occlusion in each main branch of the aorta in pulseless disease. (Sano K., Tadashi & Saito I. (1970) Angiography in pulseless disease. *Radiology*, **94**, 69.)

Treatment

The disease usually responds well in the early stages to corticosteroids though, in the later occlusive stage, anticoagulants and even vascular surgery may be required.

RELAPSING POLYCHONDRITIS

Although strictly a disease affecting the mucopolysaccharide component of ground substance, resulting in inflammation of the cartilages of the pinna, nasal septum, larynx and trachea, this may also affect the aortic valve and aortic root. In some cases, the disease presents clinically as a widespread vasculitis. Polychondritis may also be a feature of other connective tissue diseases, especially when the onset is acute.

Treatment is unsatisfactory though steroids may be of help in the acute phase.

ESSENTIAL MIXED CRYOGLOBULINAEMIA

This is a syndrome of intermittent cutaneous vasculitis associated with circulating cryoglobulins. The cryoglobulin is 'mixed' (i.e. more than one class of immunoglobulin).

Clinical features

Intermittent palpable purpura (histology—leucocytoclastic vasculitis) involving the legs.

Exacerbated by exercise and exposure to cold.

May lead to chronic ulceration.

Associated features include Raynaud's phenomenon, myalgias, arthralgias, Sjögren's syndrome, and (rarely) nephritis.

Treatment

Mild cases require no treatment. In severe cases, steroids, azathioprine or cyclophosphamide are used. Plasma exchange is effective in some cases, especially when combined with immunosuppression.

HENOCH-SCHOENLEIN (ANAPHYLACTOID) PURPURA

This is a syndrome of vasculitic purpura, arthritis, gastrointestinal, and renal lesions, usually following upper respiratory tract infections and more common in children.

The histology is that of a leucocytoclastic vasculitis, with IgA deposited both in the involved dermal vessels and in the glomerular mesangium.

Clinical features and epidemiology

Most common in 2 to 8 year olds.
Male predominance.

Preceding upper respiratory tract infection in 90%.
Fever.
Palpable purpura, especially in lower limbs and buttocks.
Colicky abdominal pain; gastrointestinal blood loss.
Transient, non-migratory polyarthritis.
Acute glomerulitis in 50% of patients.

Treatment

Disease is usually self-limiting within a month.
Severe cases require dapsone or prednisolone.

17 Polymyalgia Rheumatica and Giant Cell Arteritis

POLYMYALGIA RHEUMATICA (PMR)

A clinical syndrome characterised by pain and stiffness in the muscles of the pelvic and shoulder girdles without evidence of a primary muscle disorder.
Patients are usually over 50 years of age. ESR usually occurs over 50. There is rapid relief of symptoms within a few days with low dose corticosteroids.

GIANT CELL ARTERITIS (GCA)

A pathological entity with a number of clinical manifestations, one of which is polymyalgia rheumatica.
The cause of PMR is unknown. GCA is frequently found in patients with PMR but the mechanism by which GCA produces polymyalgic symptoms is obscure.

POLYMYALGIA RHEUMATICA

Epidemology

Prevalence   Relatively common

Age   A disorder of late-middle and old age; rare under 50.

Sex   Females to males ratio 2:1.

Pathology

Muscle biopsy is normal.
Synovitis has been found in the knees, shoulders and sternoclavicular joints.
GCA may be associated.

Clinical features

MUSCULOSKELETAL

Pain, stiffness and 'weakness':
— the onset may be insidious but is sometimes so abrupt that the patient can remember the hour at which the illness began
— distribution: the muscles of the shoulder, neck and pelvic girdles.
— true weakness is absent; severe stiffness causes functional impairment but weakness is proportional to pain
— symptoms are usually symmetrical but occasionally affect only one site and may be asymmetrical.
Mild large joint synovitis occurs occasionally.

SYSTEMIC

Changes may include:
— generalised malaise
— anorexia
— weight loss which may be marked
— fevers and night sweats. These can be severe and may present a confusing picture suggesting malignancy, infection or other connective tissue disorders.

GIANT CELL ARTERITIS

Other manifestations of giant cell or cranial arteritis may occur when GCA is associated with the polymyalgic syndrome.

Laboratory findings

ABNORMAL

ESR invariably raised, often to over 100 mm/hr.
Anaemia: normochromic, normocytic—common.
$\alpha 1$ and $\alpha 2$ globulins often increased.
Serum alkaline phosphatase is sometimes elevated.

NORMAL

Serum creatine phosphokinase.
Electromyography.

Muscle biopsy.

X-rays (although these may show degenerative changes which are common in this age group).

Rose Waaler and Latex test.

Diagnosis and differential diagnosis

Diseases which may present with a *polymyalgic* onset include:

INFECTIONS

The myalgia of viral infections may be severe but is usually short lived.

Appropriate clinical and laboratory investigations should be performed to exclude serious bacterial infections, e.g. SBE.

RHEUMATOID ARTHRITIS

May present as PMR but the development of typical peripheral joint synovitis and positive serology usually clarifies the situation.

POLYARTERITIS NODOSA

Skin involvement, renal lesions, pulmonary disease and peripheral neuropathy are absent in PMR.

PAN does not selectively involve the temporal vessels.

POLYMYOSITIS

Weakness rather than pain and stiffness is the major characteristic of polymyositis.

The typical skin rash may suggest dermatomyositis.

Evidence of primary muscle involvement indicated by a raised CPK, abnormal EMG and positive muscle biopsy is not found in PMR.

SLE

Polymyalgia may be a prominent initial symptom but typical serology usually distinguishes this condition.

It is unusual for SLE to present in old age.

GENERALISED FIBROMYALGIA

Pain and stiffness are less severe and are unaccompanied by significant systemic symptoms; the E S R is normal.

MALIGNANCY

P M R is not specifically associated with malignancy but myeloma, lymphoma and other malignancies may present with generalised aches and pains.

Lymphadenopathy and splenomegaly do not occur in P M R.

Serum and urinary protein studies will exclude myeloma.

P M R, although a diagnosis of exclusion, is now a well recognised entity. While the range of differential diagnoses should be considered clinically, unnecessary laboratory and radiological investigation of elderly patients can be avoided if the characteristic features of P M R are recognised.

Course

P M R is said to be a self-limiting disease, usually lasting 12–24 months but sometimes it persists for many years. The danger of P M R is the risk of blindness as a complication of associated giant cell arteritis.

GIANT CELL ARTERITIS

Pathology

This is an inflammatory condition of the arterial wall.

Early lesions are:
— degeneration and fragmentation of the fibres of the internal elastic lamina
— a chronic inflammatory infiltrate of lymphocytes, histiocytes and scattered foreign body giant cells containing phagocytosed elastic fibres around the internal elastic lamina
— endothelial and subendothelial fibroblast proliferation with nodular or diffuse thickening of the intima and narrowing of the lumen.

Later changes include:
— mononuclear cell infiltrate with granulomatous destruction of the media
— fibrotic changes.

These lesions are *patchy* with segments of normal artery between affected areas. The segmental distribution of the pathology reduces the frequency of positive biopsies.

Extent of pathology:
— predominantly affects the superficial temporal, ophthalmic, posterior ciliary and vertebral arteries
— other large arteries may include internal and external carotid, subclavian, brachial, abdominal arteries and aorta
— intracranial arteries are infrequently affected.

Clinical Manifestations

Common:
— polymyalgia rheumatica
— anaemia, fever, anorexia and weight loss
— headache and scalp tenderness
— visual disturbances:
  ptosis
  diplopia
  transient or permanent, partial or complete, visual loss.

Less Common:
— pain or claudication in tongue or jaw
— cerebral effects:
  aphasia, vertigo, 'stroke'
  dementia and psychosis
— peripheral
— intermittent claudication
— myocardial infarction
— aortic arch syndrome
— aortic aneurysm.

RELATIONSHIP BETWEEN PMR AND GCA AND BLINDNESS

1 In PMR, temporal artery biopsy will demonstrate GCA in:
— 15% of patients without clinical evidence of GCA
— up to 80% of patients with clinical evidence of GCA.

Since GCA is a patchy lesion, 'blind' biopsy underestimates the incidence of GCA in PMR; the actual association is therefore unknown.

Some believe that PMR is always a manifestation of GCA; most consider this unlikely.

2 In patients with GCA:
— visual disturbances are common
— 5% go blind in one or both eyes.
Transient visual disturbances commonly precede blindness.
3 In patients with PMR with a negative temporal artery biopsy, visual disturbances are rarely the initial manifestation of GCA.

MANAGEMENT OF PMR AND GCA

Polymyalgia rheumatica

1 Exclude other diagnoses.
2 Temporal artery biopsy:
— this should be performed if there is any clinical suspicion of GCA, e.g. tenderness of temporal arteries, headaches etc.
— in patients without evidence of GCA many authorities consider that it is still advisable to perform a biopsy but this is not a universal practice
— biopsy should be taken from a site of tenderness, thickening or diminished pulsation.
3 If biopsy is negative or not indicated, treat with prednisone to control symptoms:
— most patients respond to prednisolone 10–15 mgm daily with dramatic relief of symptoms
— it is advisable to begin with a low dose, increasing it only if necessary; after some weeks the dose can generally be reduced
— the ESR falls slowly; although the patient may have become asymptomatic, the ESR may take several weeks to return to normal
— treatment may have to be continued for up to 2 years; the guides to the correct maintenance dose of prednisone are control of symptoms and control of the ESR (older patients may have raised ESRs)
— treatment with too small a dose for too short a period is often associated with recurrence
— manifestations of GCA can still appear despite a negative initial biopsy and low dose steroids; patients should be warned to report any suspicious symptoms and they should be kept under surveillance.
There has been a tendency to over treat some cases because of the well known risk of blindness. In older patients, the risks of steroid

side effects such as osteoporosis may have to be balanced against the need to bring the E S R down to normal.

4   If biopsy shows changes of G C A; treat the G C A.

Giant cell arteritis

1   If G C A is suspected clinically:
—   commence steroids immediately with prednisone 40–60 mgm daily. Temporal artery biopsy should be done as soon as possible but, in view of the risk of blindness, steroid therapy should not be delayed.
—   high dose steroid should be continued for 1 to 3 months and then slowly reduced.

2   Blindness in G C A:
—   although steroids have substantially reduced the incidence of blindness, visual impairment and blindness can occur in patients on corticosteroids
—   management: steroid dose should be increased to 80 mgm daily and anticoagulation commenced with heparin (providing there are no contraindications).

18 Crystal-induced Arthropathies

It has long been recognised that monosodium urate crystals cause gout. In recent years, it has become evident that other crystals may also cause arthritis (Table 18.1).

The major crystal-induced arthropathies are due to:

1 Monosodium urate crystals (urate) which cause acute gout and chronic tophaceous gout.

2 Calcium pyrophosphate crystals which cause acute pseudogout and other chronic arthropathies.

Other crystals which may cause arthritis include:

3 Crystalised injected corticosteriod which cause acute synovitis.

4 Calcium hydroxyapatite crystals which cause acute calcific periarthritis and possibly cause acute synovitis in osteoarthritis.

PATHOGENESIS OF CRYSTAL-INDUCED SYNOVITIS

Important crystal characteristics

Size. Aggregates or individual crystals $<20\,\mu$m are most inflammatory.

Surface. Presentation of positively charged hydrogen atoms promote bonding with complementary negatively charged groups such as those on proteins and phospholipids. Surface binding of immunoglobulin promotes phagocytosis through the Fc receptors on polymorphonuclear leucocytes.

Phagocytosis

Phagocytosis of crystals by polymorphonuclear leucocytes is critical to the development of an inflammatory response. Mononuclear and synovial lining cells also ingest crystals.

Typically, cells ingest particles such as crystals within a

Table 18.1 Synovial fluid crystals

Crystal	Size μm	Shape	Birefringence	Comment
Monosodium urate	2–20	Rod or needle	Strongly negative	May be intracellular
Calcium pyrophosphate	2–25	Rhomboidal, blunt needle or irregular	Weakly positive	May be intracellular
Crystalised corticosteroid	1–20	Irregular: rods, granules or debris	Strongly positive or negative	May be intracellular
Cholesterol	Often >100	Flat rhomboidal plates; occasional needle	Negative	Never intracellular
Dicalcium phosphate dihydrate			Positive	? role in joint disease
Artifacts:				
calcium oxalate	2–10	Variable	Positive	May be intracellular
lithium heparin	2–5	Maltese cross	Positive	May be intracellular
glove powder	Variable			

membranous sac (*phagosome*) which fuses with the enzyme-rich lysosome to digest the crystal within a phagolysosome.

Phagocytosed pyrophosphate crystals are typically seen within a phagolysosomal sac; by contrast, urate crystals are not usually enclosed within a phagosome.

Membrane Lysis and Enzyme Release

Urate crystals cause damage to membranes more quickly and efficiently than calcium pyrophosphate, probably because of their hydrogen bonding characteristics.

Phagolysosomal lysis results in the release of enzymes into the cell cytoplasm; in gout, cytoplasmic enzymes are also released from the cell, indicating loss of integrity of the cell membrane.

Further Chemotaxis and Inflammation

Crystal phagocytosis by polymorphonuclear leucocytes is followed by the release of a chemotactic factor; this effect is partially blocked by colchicine following urate crystal ingestion.

Other chemotactic factors may be generated by complement components activated by urate crystals.

More polymorphonuclear leucocytes promote further crystal phagocytosis and the release of further lysosomal enzymes.

The coagulation, kinin, plasmin and complement systems may all be involved in further inflammatory activity.

CRYSTAL IDENTIFICATION

Definitive crystal identification may require sophisticated techniques such as X-ray diffraction analysis or chemical analysis. For routine clinical purposes the standard technique to identify crystals in synovial fluid is compensated polarised light microscopy.

Polarised light microscopy

Light is polarised when it is orientated and aligned in one plane; the addition of a second polariser rotated at 90° to the first will block light and produce a black background. If crystals are placed between crossed polarisers they diffract the light rays so that they pass through the second polariser and produce a bright image of the crystal on a black background. Materials which diffract light in this way are said to be birefringent.

Compensated polarised light microscopy

When a 'first order red filter' or compensator is placed between the crystal and the first polariser a pink or rose-coloured background is produced and the crystals appear yellow or blue. The compensator allows further crystal identification because different crystals show different optical characteristics with respect to their orientation to the axis of the compensator.

When the axis of the crystal is parallel to the axis of the compensator:

— positively birefringent crystals are blue
— negatively birefringent crystals are yellow.

When the axis of the crystal is at 90° to the axis of the compensator:

— positively birefringent crystals are yellow
— negatively birefringent crystals are blue.

The characteristics of crystals and other birefringent material which may be seen in the synovial fluid are shown in Table 18.1.

19 Gout

Gout is an inflammatory arthritis resulting from the deposition of urate crystals in and around joints. The development of urate crystalisation in gout almost invariably requires a high serum level of uric acid.

HISTORY

Gout is one of medicine's best documented diseases, beloved by medical historians. Urate has been identified in the great toe of an Egyptian mummy and was referred to in some detail by Hippocrates, who, amongst his other aphorisms noted that women did not suffer from gout until the menopause. Garrod noted that the blood of gout subjects contained an excess of sodium urate. This century has seen the detailed study of some of the enzyme defects associated with gout and the discovery of allopurinol, which has revolutionised treatment.

EPIDEMIOLOGY

Prevalence Figures vary from 1–20 per 1000 males. Gout is generally commoner amongst affluent societies. In certain groups, such as some Polynesian islanders, there is a strikingly high prevalence where strong evidence for hereditory factors has emerged.

Sex and age Before the age of 50, primary gout is a male disease. Acute gout in a pre-menopausal female is so rare that the diagnosis of secondary gout must be assumed until proved otherwise. Gout is rare below the age of 30 except in those individuals with enzyme defects. The peak age of first attacks in males is 40–50 and in post-menopausal females 50–60. Some 50% of individuals with primary gout have a positive family history.

CLINICAL FEATURES

Acute gout

In 70–90% of individuals, the initial attack of gout affects the big toe; podagra is the term applied to acute gout affecting the first MTP joint. The pain often develops at night. It may follow local trauma to the joint, or may occur at the site of an old injury. One characteristic presentation of gout is following stress, such as an operation or acute illness such as a coronary thrombosis. Within hours, there is intense pain, swelling and redness. The pain may become so severe that bedclothes cannot be tolerated against the joint. Constitutional features such as fever are rare. The attack may settle spontaneously in days or weeks, though more commonly is aborted by therapy.

A second attack may follow within days, but, alternatively may not occur for many years, or ever. For this reason, long-term therapy is generally not advised following an isolated attack (*see* p. 206).

After the big toe, other joints most frequently affected by acute gout are the ankle, knees, fingers, elbows and wrists. The spine is rarely if ever affected in acute gout. Polyarticular acute gout occurs rarely.

PREDISPOSING FACTORS

Acute gout is almost always associated with long standing hyperuricaemia.
Other predisposing factors include:
— drugs, especially diuretics
— local stress (e.g. a blow to the joint)
— post operative stress
— medical stress, e.g. myocardial infarction
— during the institution of allopurinol therapy (*see later*)
— gross over indulgence in food (e.g. seafood) or alcohol.

Chronic gout

In the days before adequate treatment, and nowadays mostly in non-compliant patients or some with metabolic defects, acute attacks become more frequent, ultimately leading to chronic polyarthritis. Urate crystals coat, then damage the joint cartilage and deposits of urate (tophus) form within the joint. Later, especially in the small joints of the hands and feet, tophaceous deposits in and around the joint result in permanent destructive joint damage and deformity (Fig. 19.1).

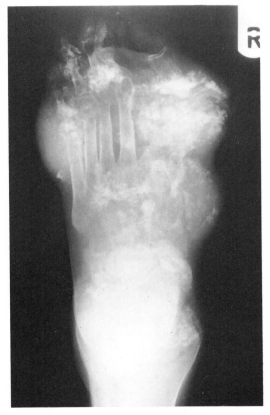

Fig. 19.1A   Severe gout. Widespread tophi and joint destruction. (Hughes G.R., Barnes C.G., & Mason R.M. (1968) Bony alkylosis in Gout. *Annals of Rheumatic Disease* **27**, 67.)

A characteristic late radiological appearance is of erosions, overlaid by soft tissue swelling; and often containing secondary calcific deposits.

A common feature of chronic gout is olecranon bursitis.

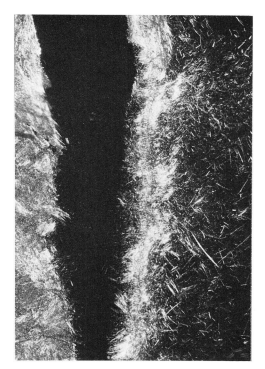

Fig. 19.1B   Articular cartilage in gout showing urate crystals. (Hughes G.R., Barnes C.G., & Mason R.M., (1968) Bony alkylosis in Gout. *Annals of Rheumatic Disease* **27,** 67.)

TOPHUS

The presence of tophi usually reflects severe untreated gout. They are deposits of urate, at first solid, but later softening and containing chalky material. They form as small nodules in cartilaginous sites—particularly on the helix of the ear and around joint cartilage, and around tendons. Other sites include the kidney (*see* p. 202), bursae, and, rarely, in viscera such as the heart, pleura, and meninges.

Small tophi remain intact as discreet, subcutaneous nodes. As they enlarge, the overlying skin becomes smooth and shiny, finally ulcerating to discharge moist chalky white material.

Treatment with allopurinol usually results in a reduction of size of tophi.

KIDNEY DISEASE

Renal stones. Urate calculi occur in approximately 5% of gout patients. Uric acid stones form particularly in acid urine (e.g. common after ileostomies where urinary pH values are low). They are translucent on X-ray and may occur in the absence of hyperuricaemia. Multiple renal stones may ultimately lead to obstruction, infection and renal failure.

Gouty kidney. Rarely patients with long-standing tophaceous gout may develop proteinuria, decreased creatinine clearance and hypertension. This form of renal impairment is thought to be due to widespread deposits of urate in the interstitial tissues.

Hypertension. Hypertension (diastolic pressure over 90 mmHg) is found in up to one-third of gout patients and may contribute to renal impairment. The reasons for this association are not clear.

OTHER DISEASE ASSOCIATIONS

In addition to hypertension, there is an increased incidence of diabetes and ischaemic heart disease in gout patients—indeed ischaemia is a far more frequent cause of death than renal failure. One possible link is the increased incidence of Type IV hyperlipoproteinaemia and other lipid abnormalities seen in these patients.

HYPERURICAEMIA

A far commoner problem than clinical gout is the finding of idiopathic hyperuricaemia. Indeed with the advent of widespread blood screening for insurance and other purposes, the significance of hyperuricaemia, and its management, are important topics.

The widely accepted normal mean upper limit of uric acid in blood is 7 mg% (0.42 mmol/l) in man and 5 mg% (0.30 mmol/l) for women. Hyperuricaemia is divided into primary and secondary. Causes of hyperuricaemia are listed in Table 19.1.

Primary hyperuricaemia

In the majority of cases, the aetiology of hyperuricaemia is multifactorial. The following factors may each contribute:
— genetic
— family history

Table 19.1 Causes of hyperuricaemia

Hyperuricaemia	Causes
Primary	Aetiology usually unknown A small number of cases where an enzyme defect is demonstrated (Lesch–Nyhan syndrome)

Secondary	Haemopoietic:
	  myeloproliferative disorders
	  polycythaemia
	  large tumors
	  irradiation
	
	Drugs:
	  thiazides (the single commonest cause)
	  most diuretics
	  low dose aspirin
	  pyrazinamide
	  cytotoxic agents
	
	Metabolic:
	  ketosis and starvation
	  hyperlipidaemia
	  fructose administration
	  lactic acid anaemia
	
	Renal:
	  renal impairment
	  decreased urine flow
	  association with hypertension
	
	Miscellaneous:
	  myxoedema
	  hypercalcaemia
	  psoriasis
	  lead poisoning
	  sarcoidosis
	  excessive purine or alcohol intake
	  obesity

— hypertension
— hypertriglyceridaemia
— alcohol and purine intake
— stress
— dehydration
— mild renal impairment
— obesity.
In a small number of cases, enzyme defects have been demon-

strated. The well-known example is the rare disease, Lesch-Nyhan syndrome.

LESCH-NYHAN SYNDROME

The pathways leading to uric acid formation are shown in Figure 19.2. The enzyme hypoxanthine-guanine-phosphoribosyltransferase (HGPRT) is responsible for the utilisation of the purine

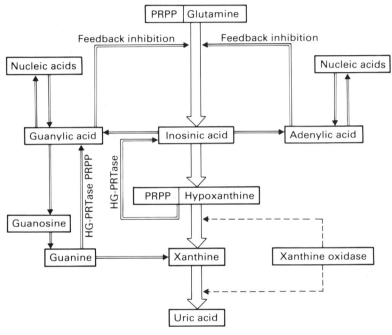

PRPP = 5-phosphoribosyl-l-pyrophosphate
HG-PRTase = hypoxanthine-guaninephosphoribosyltransferase

Fig. 19.2   Pathways of uric acid formation.

bases hypoxanthine and guanine. A defect in this enzyme results in severe overproduction of uric acid. Mild degrees of deficiency of this enzyme result in a severe excess production of urate. In the most severe form (the Lesch–Nyhan Syndrome) there is severe mental impairment, choreiform movements, spasticity, and a bizarre form of self-mutilation.

OTHER ENZYME DISORDERS

Other important enzymes used in the degradation of nucleic acids include phosphoribosyl-pyrophosphate (PRPP) synthetase, a defect of which also results in excess urate production.

Secondary hyperuricaemia

Serum uric acid levels are a result of the balance between production and excretion. Purines are produced in most cells, notably those of the liver. Cell death results in the formation of purine bases and uric acid. The final degradation of purine bases to uric acid is dependent on xanthine oxidase, an enzyme particularly concentrated in liver, bone marrow and intestinal mucosal cells. In myeloproliferative diseases such as leukaemia, where degradation of bone marrow cells occurs, an excess production of uric acid occurs.

Two-thirds of urate is eliminated via the urine. Normal urine

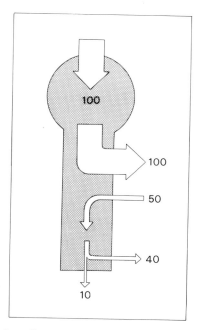

Fig. 19.3   Filtration of urate.

urate excretion is less than 600 mg per 24 hours (36 mmol/24-hours) in individuals on purine-free diets. In the kidney, it is thought that 100% of urate is filtered, almost 100% reabsorbed in the proximal tubule, about 50% actively re-secreted in the distal tubule and, finally 10% excreted in the urine (Fig. 19.3). Thus drugs and metabolic influences on the renal tubules, as well as on cell breakdown, have a general effect on serum uric acid levels.

DIAGNOSIS

In classical, acute podagra, diagnosis is easy. Although proof of diagnosis, in theory, requires the microscopic demonstration of intracellular urate crystals in a synovial fluid aspirate, this is rarely undertaken as the aspiration of a small joint in an acutely inflamed toe is almost impossibly painful.

The main differential diagnosis of a 'hot, red joint' is septic arthritis.

Points favouring a diagnosis of gout:
— previous attacks
— typical clinical picture includes rapid onset
— relative lack of systemic features
— response to high dose NSAID
— hyperuricaemia (in practice, the result is usually unavailable in time to be helpful)

Points favouring septic arthritis:
— slower onset
— accompanying fever, chills, malaise
— site of entry of infection
— leucocytosis

Gout is overdiagnosed. The patient with joint pains and mild or even moderate hyperuricaemia may well have an unrelated disorder, such as seronegative arthritis or osteoarthritis with hyperuricaemia resulting from concomitant drug therapy.

MANAGEMENT

It is essential to recognise that management involves two quite separate issues:
1 Treatment of acute gout.
2 Evaluation and management of hyperuricaemia.

Acute Gout

The treatment of choice is indomethacin, phenylbutazone or one of the newer NSAID.

The most important factor in effective treatment is speed of NSAID administration; treatment should be started in high dose as early as possible in the attack.

Indomethacin

Usually given with food in divided doses up to 200 mg on the first day and 25–50 mg tds thereafter. If side effects such as headache, nausea or vomiting are a problem, alternative preparations such as slow release indomethacin (75 mg) or suppositories may be used.

Phenylbutazone

Arguably the best drug for acute gout but its marrow depressing effect (exceptionally rare in short term administration) has caused this drug to be withdrawn in many countries.

Azapropazone

300 mgm qds is proving a very useful third alternative.

Colchicine

Traditionally the treatment for acute gout, is limited in its usefulness by its tendency to cause nausea and diarrhoea, often before the therapeutic effect is achieved. The traditional dose is 1 mg orally followed by 0.5 mg every 2 hours until the gout is controlled or intolerable side effects occur.

Intra-articular steroids

Provide the quickest relief in an acute attack and this approach is indicated in large joint involvement.

Once the acute attack has settled, the patient's uric acid 'status' should be evaluated. However, *during* the attack, the serum uric acid should not be reduced, since this may exacerbate and prolong the acute synovitis.

Asymptomatic Hyperuricaemia—Evaluation

Hyperuricaemia should not be diagnosed on the basis of a single serum uric acid level which can be influenced by many factors.

Whether hyperuricaemia is detected in the asymptomatic individual or in patients with acute or chronic tophaceous gout, the evaluation process is the same:

1 Repeat the serum uric acid; fasting, perhaps on several occasions.

2 Eliminate drugs which are unnecessary but may affect urate levels:
— ascorbic acid may spuriously alter laboratory urate reading
— low dose aspirin, a high purine diet and alcohol may transiently elevate serum urate levels.

3 Perform a full clinical assessment looking for:
— conditions which increase urate levels such as obesity, myeloproliferative conditions, renal impairment
— conditions which may result from chronic hyperuricaemia such as renal stones and nephropathy
— conditions associated with hyperuricaemia such as hyperlipidaemia, hypertension, etc.

4 Undertake relevant investigations including:
— full blood count, lipid profile, biochemistry
— renal function including urinalysis, urea, creatinine, electrolytes and creatinine clearance with radiological evaluation, if indicated
— urinary uric acid to determine whether the patient is overproducing or under-excreting relative to serum urate levels.

Management of Hyperuricaemia

METHODS OF SERUM URATE REDUCTION

Nonpharmacological measures:
— weight reduction
— increased urine flow by increased (nonalcoholic) fluid intake
— avoidance of alcohol and drugs which elevate urate levels, e.g. low dose aspirin
— low purine diet.

Drugs:

Allopurinol
A xanthine oxidase inhibitor which blocks the enzyme which converts hypoxanthine to xanthine
Dose: it is advisable to begin with a low dose, e.g. 100 mgm daily slowly increasing over a period of weeks or months to the maintenance dose, i.e. the dose which maintains the serum uric acid

level within the normal range; this is generally around 300–600 mgm daily
— in patients with reduced creatinine clearance, the maintenance dose should be reduced.

Side effects: unusual but may be severe and serious; they include skin rashes, hypersensitivity reactions, bone marrow depression and cholestasis
— in common with any agent lowering the serum urate the most frequent side effect is the precipitation of acute gout
— an important interaction involves azathioprine which may be potentiated by allopurinol since azathioprine is normally metabolised by xanthine oxidase.

Uricosuric drugs
Used less frequently, they include
— probenecid which inhibits tubular reabsorption of urate, usual dose is 1–2 G bd with liberal fluid and a urinary alkaliser
— sulphinpyrazone 100–200 mgm bd
— azapropazone which has both anti-inflammatory and uricosuric effects.

Since serum urate lowering drugs may precipitate acute gout, it is advisable that their introduction be 'covered' by
— colchicine 0.5 mgm bd or tds, or
— indomethacin 25 mgm bd or tds
and that these be continued until the serum urate is stable within the normal range.

Note: if acute gout occurs *during* maintenance therapy
— do not stop drug
— treat acute attack
— re-evaluate adequency of maintenance dose once attack has settled.

APPROACH TO HYPERURICAEMIA

If an individual is found to be truly and persistently hyperuricaemic further management will depend on the clinical setting and, to a lesser extent, the serum urate level.

Asymptomatic hyperuricaemia:
— in the majority of patients, nonpharmacological measures only are required

— the patient should be observed and the urate level checked from time to time, e.g. six-monthly
— if the serum urate is above 9 mgm% or 0.55 mmol/l, some authorities would advocate prophylactic drug treatment.

Hyperuricaemia with intermittent acute gout:
— a single attack of acute gout is generally insufficient basis on which to commence drug therapy
— if two or more attacks have occurred and hyperuricaemia cannot be controlled by simpler measures, drug therapy, usually allopurinol, is indicated
— logically, if the clinical situation justifies drugs, therapy must be lifelong; hence the need to consider their introduction carefully.

Hyperuricaemia with chronic tophaceous gout or renal calculi:
— the need to control urate levels is clearcut and drug therapy is usually necessary.

Chronic Tophaceous Gout

Management usually includes:
— drug therapy of hyperuricaemia together with simpler measures
— intermittent treatment of intervening acute attacks of gout
— long-term NSAID administration for control of symptoms arising from chronic joint damage.

PROGNOSIS

The advent of allopurinol has meant that, in theory, the patient should remain free of acute attacks of gout for the remainder of his life. Urate nephrolithiasis and 'gouty kidney' are no longer a significant cause of mortality in most gout patients. The major causes of death remains hypertensive and atheromatous vascular disease. The former is treatable. The overall prognosis for vascular disease in gouty patients may improve if the lipid abnormalities seen in association with gout are detected and treated as a matter of routine at the time the gout itself is diagnosed.

20 Calcium Pyrophosphate Deposition Disease

Calcium pyrophosphate deposition disease (CPPD) is, after gout, the second most common crystal-induced arthritis. Confusion has arisen with respect to some terms used to describe aspects of the disease, e.g. *pseudogout* is one clinical manifestation of CPPD—an acute inflammatory arthritis resembling gout. *Chrondrocalcinosis* refers to the presence of calcium pyrophosphate (CPPi) crystals in articular cartilage and can be detected only on X-ray or histological examination of cartilage.

EPIDEMIOLOGY

Prevalence Symptomatic CPPD is about a half to a third as common as gout. Chondrocalcinosis is detected in about 5% of the adult population but in a considerably higher percentage of old people.

Sex Male to female ratio is 1–2:1.

Age Familial forms—early onset; sporadic forms—onset in sixth or seventh decade.

CLASSIFICATION

Hereditary forms: Czech, Dutch, and Spanish:	<1%
Associated with metabolic diseases:	5%
Idiopathic—most common:	>90%

AETIOLOGY AND PATHOLOGY

Calcium pyrophosphate crystal formation

Calcium pyrophosphate crystals are found only in articular cartilage and some closely associated tissues such as synovium and surrounding ligamentous and tendinous structures.

In the idiopathic form there is no evidence that calcium pyrophosphate crystal formation is due to a systemic metabolic disturbance. Although a variety of biosynthetic reactions produce pyrophosphate, no enzyme deficiencies have been recognised in patients with CPPD.

It is thought likely that local factors in cartilage favour calcium pyrophosphate deposition.

Crystal induction of inflammation

Unlike gout, in which urate crystals precipitate from super-saturated synovial fluid, calcium pyrophosphate crystals are thought to enter the joint cavity after being 'shed' from cartilage in which they have formed.

The mechanism by which they then produce inflammation is outlined in Chapter 17.

CLINICAL MANIFESTATIONS

It is well recognised the CPPD causes or is associated with several different clinical entities.

Pseudogout

Acute inflammatory arthritis resembling gout.
Males affected more commonly than females.
Attacks commonly precipitated by:
— surgery
— medical illnesses
— trauma.
Sites:
— knee most common
— also other large joints: shoulders, ankles, wrists, hips, occasionally small joints of feet.
Typical attack:
— onset over $\frac{1}{2}$–$2\frac{1}{2}$days
— occasionally follows stress (e.g. surgery, coronary thrombosis)
— one of the major causes of acute monoarthritis in the elderly
— generally monoarticular, occasionally oligoarticular with involvement of one or more neighbouring joints in a 'cluster' attack
— lasts $\frac{1}{2}$–30 days; averages about 9 days.
Mild attacks also occur with transient pains, stiffness and slight effusion.

Pseudo-osteoarthritis with or without acute episodes

CPPD is commonly associated with degenerative arthritis which is punctuated by intermittent acute episodes in about 50%.
Females affected more commonly than males.
Sites:
— knees, wrists, MCP joints, hips, shoulders, elbows, ankles
— generally symmetrical.
Flexion contractions are common.
Chondrocalcinosis may or may not be seen on X-ray.
This type of degenerative arthritis differs from primary osteoarthritis in several respects:
— joint distribution: wrists, MCP, shoulders and ankle joints not involved in primary OA
— X-ray may show prominent subchondral cyst formation, severe destructive changes and prominent hook osteophytes at the MCP joints as well as chandrocalcinosis.

Asymptomatic CPPD

Probably the most common type.
Chrondrocalcinosis detected on X-ray.

Pseudorheumatoid arthritis

A rare entity.
Symmetrical, rheumatoid arthritis-like inflammatory polyarthritis.
Rheumatoid factor typically negative.

Pseudoneuropathic arthritis

Very rarely, CPPD occurs in association with a markedly destructive arthropathy of Charcot type.
Possibly Charcot joints are most likely to develop in patients with neuropathy who also have CPPD.

DISEASES ASSOCIATED WITH CPPD

CPPD has been reported in association with a large number of diseases. Since it is a common disorder, the likelihood of a true association with other common disorders, such as diabetes and hypertension, has been questioned.

Diseases in which true association is likely:

1 Hyperparathyroidism:
— about 20% of patients with hyperparathyroidism have CPPD
— it is claimed that up to 5% of patients with CPPD have hyperparathyroidism.

2 Haemochromatosis:
— 40–45% of patients with haemochromatosis have CPPD.

3 Hypothyroidism.

4 Gout.

5 Other rare conditions:
— hypophosphatasia
— hypomagnesemia
— Wilson's disease.

DIAGNOSIS

Diagnosis is based on radiology and synovial fluid analysis.

Radiology

CHONDROCALCINOSIS

Calcification of hyaline cartilage produces a fine line parallel to joint surface (Fig. 20.1).

Calcification of fibrocartilage produces a stippled or punctate opacity and is commonly seen in the menisci of the knee and the triangular cartilage of the wrists.

Chondrocalcinosis is most likely to be seen in the knee, symphysis pubis and wrist.

Calcification may also occur in articular capsules.

DEGENERATIVE ARTHRITIS

Often involving sites which are not affected by primary osteoarthritis: wrists, MCP, shoulders, etc.

Characterised by large subchondral cysts, osteophytosis and marked destructive changes.

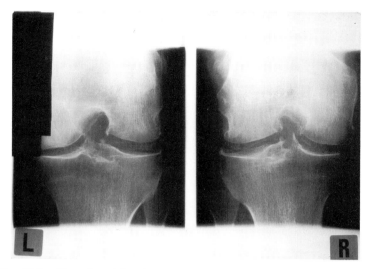

Fig. 20.1 Chondrocalcinosis.

Synovial fluid analysis

DURING ACUTE SYNOVITIS

High white cell count.
Calcium pyrophosphate crystals shown on compensated polarised light microscopy (*see* Chapter 17).
Crystals are:
— 2-25 μm long
— rhomboidal, occasionally needle shaped with a blunt end
— weakly positively birefringent
— often intracellular.

DURING CHRONIC EFFUSION

Crystals may be found in synovial fluid even when there are few white cells.

Routine biochemistry

In idiopathic CPPD, routine biochemistry is normal although elderly patients may show:
— rheumatoid factor in about 5%

— hyperuricaemia in about 5%
— impaired glucose tolerance.
In secondary CPPD the biochemical abnormalities of the associated disease may be evident, e.g. hyperparathyroidism.

MANAGEMENT

There is no treatment for CPPD comparable to allopurinol in hyperuricaemia and gout. It is not possible to remove calcium pyrophosphate from tissues or prevent its continued deposition.

Acute synovitis: pseudogout

Aspiration of synovial fluid followed by intra-articular injection of corticosteroid. Relief is usually dramatic.
Non-steroidal anti-inflammatory drugs, e.g. indomethacin, are effective; colchicine has a more variable effect than in acute gout.

Chronic arthropathy

Treat as for osteoarthritis.
For badly damaged joints—prosthetic replacement surgery may be indicated.

Associated diseases

Treatment of hyperparathyroidism and haemochromatosis is not known to effect the deposition of calcium pyrophosphate or alter CPPD.
Parathyroidectomy may precipitate pseudogout.

HYDROXYAPATITE DEPOSITION DISEASE

Hydroxyapatite crystals are too small to be identified on light microscopy although they may be seen as aggregates. They have been found in synovial fluid during episodes of synovitis in osteoarthritis and in experimental models have been shown capable of producing an inflammatory response.

Calcium hydroxyapatite crystals cause acute calcific periarthritis and it is possible that they are responsible for the more inflammatory episodes which sometimes occur during the course of osteoarthritis. How often they produce clinically significant pathology remains to be determined.

21   Osteoarthritis

Osteoarthritis (OA) or degenerative joint disease is a common, chronic arthropathy characterised by 'wearing out' of the joint. The initial changes occur in the articular cartilage and the disease is usually classified into two groups

1   Primary osteoarthritis, when the cause is unknown.
2   Secondary osteoarthritis, when degeneration results from malalignment of the articular surfaces or damaged joint components.

PATHOLOGY

Normal cartilage consists of chondrocytes, a matrix of collagen and aggregated proteoglycans, and water. *Collagen* forms a tight network which contains the large proteoglycan molecules and water and provides the tensile properties of cartilage. At the articular surface, it forms a limiting membrane. *Proteoglycans* are composed of glycosaminoglycans (chondroitin sulphate and keratan sulphate) attached to a protein core with a molecular weight of $1-3 \times 10^6$. Proteoglycans are in turn attached to hyaluronic acid by a protein 'link' to form even larger aggregates which are trapped within the collagen net and so provide the resilience and stiffness of cartilage. *Water* constitutes about 70% of cartilage.

When a load is applied, the fluid pressure within the cartilage rises immediately but the cartilage deforms gradually because the water, impeded by the large proteoglycan molecules, flows out slowly.

Changes in osteoarthritis

1   Focal areas of cartilage show increased water content with increased extractability of proteoglycans.
2   Surface cartilage splits or 'fibrillates'; surrounding cartilage shows loss of proteoglycans and water.
3   Cartilage erosions develop focally, denuding the underlying

bone which becomes worn, compressed, and smooth—a process called *eburnation*.

4 Subchondral cysts form, probably as a result of synovial fluid being forced into exposed bone.

5 Osteophytes, which are bony outgrowths, occur around the joint margin.

6 Joint instability may develop as a result of capsular laxity, collapse of subchondral cysts in a weight-bearing area and muscular wasting.

7 An effusion and synovial inflammation, with non-specific histological changes, may occur secondary to trauma or the irritation of degenerative joint constituents, such as hydroxyapatite crystals.

AETIOLOGY

Primary osteoarthritis

The cause is unknown. Factors which have been considered important include:

Ageing.   Osteoarthritis is more common in the elderly but since it may begin in relatively young individuals and is not universal in the old, it cannot be considered a 'normal' ageing process.

Wear of cartilage.   Joints repetitively moved within the normal range fail to develop OA in animal models. By contrast, small impulsive forces exerted *across* the joint will rapidly lead to degenerative changes. These 'impulse forces' are normally absorbed by reflex muscular joint flexion and extension; if these shock absorption reflexes are impaired, the joint becomes subject to mechanical trauma which could lead to OA. The muscular weakness and slowing of reflexes which occurs with ageing may be relevant in this context.

Wear of bone.   The subchondral bone is also an important shock absorber. Microfractures of the trabeculae are known to occur in periarticular bone and it is thought that the continuous process of fracture and healing by microcallus formation leads to stiffening of subchondral bone, further loss of shock absorption, and increased cartilage damage.

Obesity.   Although obesity is often considered important, its role as a primary aetiological factor is unclear. While it seems logical that weight contributes to joint wear, it is difficult to explain the constant finding that the ankle joint is spared in primary OA.

Diet. There is no evidence of its relevance in OA.

Metabolic. Recognised metabolic disturbances predisposing to OA are listed under the causes of secondary OA.

Genetic. Heberden's nodes and primary generalised OA are often familial and tend to occur particularly in women. Patterns of occurrence consistent with either recessive or dominant inheritance have been reported.

Secondary osteoarthritis

Any condition causing malalignment of the articular surfaces or damage or alteration to the constituents of the joint—the bone, cartilage, capsule, ligaments or synovium—may result in accelerated wear and the development of OA. These include:

Trauma
— intra-articular fracture
— malalignment of fracture
— unequal leg lengths
— occupational, e.g. ankles in footballers, elbows and wrists in jackhammer operators.

Genetic, congenital and developmental
— hypermobility
— Ehlers–Danlos syndrome, Marfan's syndrome, etc.
— bone and cartilage dysplasias
— congenital dislocation of the hip
— Perthes' disease
— slipped femoral epiphysis.

Post-inflammatory
— septic arthritis
— rheumatoid arthritis and other inflammatory arthropathies
— gout and pseudogout.

Haemorrhagic
— haemophilia.

Metabolic and endocrine
— haemochromatosis
— ochronosis

— chondrocalcinosis
— hyperparathyroidism
— acromegaly.

Bone disorders
— aseptic necrosis
— Paget's disease.

Neuropathic (Charcot joint).

EPIDEMIOLOGY

Prevalence   Radiological changes of OA are almost universal in people over 65. Symptomatic OA is common and increases in frequency with advancing age.

Sex   In primary generalised OA, females are affected more than males.

Age   Primary OA of the hands may develop late in the fourth decade; peak age of onset is 45–60. Primary OA in weight-bearing joints usually over 40 years. Secondary OA occurs at any age depending on the cause and its severity.

SYMPTOMS

Pain
— gradual onset
— initially occurs after using the affected joint, e.g. a long walk
— in advanced disease, pain at rest becomes more common and it may be troublesome at night.

Stiffness
— common but not as severe or as prolonged as in inflammatory arthritis
— morning stiffness may last 5–15 minutes
— stiffness after immobility, e.g. in the hip, is often severe but transient.

Functional impairment
— variable
— may occur early in the hands even with little pain
— may be almost absent despite marked changes.
Systemic symptoms are not a feature of primary OA.

SIGNS

Swelling. Due to bony enlargement (*osteophyte*) or effusion.

Muscle wasting. Often early and accentuates the appearance of joint swelling.

Tenderness. Prominent in early OA of the hands and during acute exacerbations which are often associated with mild synovial inflammation.

Limitation of movement. Increases with advancing disease.

Crepitus. Usually evident in affected large joints. The traditional distinction between fine crepitus in inflammatory arthritis and coarse crepitus in degenerative disease is not clear cut and is of doubtful clinical value.

Deformity. Results from progressive disorganisation of the articular surfaces, ligamentous laxity, and muscle wasting.

JOINT INVOLVEMENT

Distribution

Joints most commonly affected include:
— spine: particularly the cervical and lumbar regions
— hands: DIP joints (Herberden's nodes), PIP joints (Bouchard's nodes), carpometacarpal joint of the thumb
— hips
— knees
— feet: first MTP joints particularly.
Joints not affected in primary OA:
— shoulders
— elbows
— wrists
— MCP joints
— ankle joints.

Patterns

Primary generalised OA:
— DIP and PIP joints commonly affected
— polyarticular involvement especially hips and knees.

Secondary OA:

Associated with a recognised predisposing cause:
— number of joints affected is determined by the cause
— may involve any joints including those which are not normally affected by primary OA, e.g., wrists, shoulders or elbows.

Features of individual joints

SPINE

Degenerative disease of the spine is considered separately in Chapter 22.

HANDS (Fig. 21.1)

Heberdens nodes may develop as inflamed and painful swelling of the DIP joints:
— acute phase settles over a few months to leave residual bony enlargement with mild to moderate pain, often exacerbated by wet, humid or changing weather
— onset may be gradual without obvious inflammation

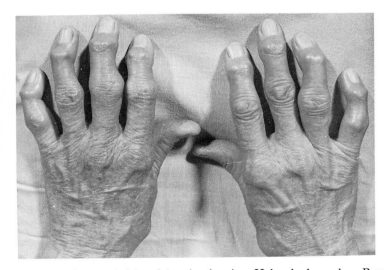

Fig. 21.1 Osteoarthritis of hands showing Hebreden's nodes, Bouchard's nodes, carpometacarpal involvement with squaring of the hand and adduction of the 1st metacarpal.

— affected joints sometimes cause lateral deviation of the distal phalanx.

Bouchard's nodes are similar to Heberden's nodes but occur at the PIP joint:

— during the inflammatory phase, prominent soft tissue swelling may cause confusion with inflammatory synovitis such as RA.

Carpometacarpal joint involvement at the thumb may cause severe pain and functional impairment (a common site for solitary OA):

— adduction of the first metacarpal bone produces a 'squared' appearance of the hand.

Interphalangeal joint of the thumb may also develop OA.

HIP JOINT

Pain usually felt maximally in the groin, thigh, buttock, lumbar region (from muscle strain) or occasionally in the knee only (referred pain via the obturator nerve):

— worse on walking and rising from a chair
— may be very severe.

Examination may reveal:

— a limp
— hip held in flexion and external rotation
— positive Trendelenberg test
— leg shortening
— limitation of movement especially extension and internal rotation
— muscle wasting of glutei and quadriceps.

X-rays: in the symptomatic patient, radiological changes are usually consistent with the degree of clinical severity.

KNEE JOINT

Both the tibiofemoral joint and the patellofemoral joint may be affected by OA.

Pain:

— of the tibiofemoral OA is felt deep in the knee or around the tibial joint margin or upper tibia
— of patellofemoral OA is felt behind the patella and is noticed particularly on ascending or descending stairs.

Instability and weakness is common in advanced disease; if loose bodies are present, the knee may lock or give way.

Examination may reveal:
— bony enlargement around the joint margin
— fixed flexion or limitation of movement
— knee joint or patellofemoral crepitus
— effusion; during an acute exacerbation, the knee may feel warm
— Baker's cyst (*see* p. 45)
— quadriceps wasting
— deformity: valgus or varus deformity with varying degrees of collateral or cruciate ligament instability.

FEET

First MTP joint very commonly affected:
— pain may be severe
— the joint may become immobile (hallux rigidus)
— hallux valgus deformity is commonly associated; this predisposes to painful bursitis over the medial surface of the joint (bunion).

Subtalar and midtarsal joints sometimes affected:
— pain and tenderness occur in the midfoot or dorsum.

LABORATORY TESTS

Routine laboratory tests are normal in primary OA.
Haematology
Hb and WCC: normal
ESR: normal; a borderline elevation sometimes seen during exacerbations especially in obese women.
Rheumatoid factor
Negative.
Biochemical profile
Normal.
Synovial fluid
Non-inflammatory
— clear, straw-coloured
— viscosity high
— WCC is usually less than 1000 cmm, occasionally to 2000 cmm during acute flare
— predominantly mononuclear cells.

RADIOLOGY

The X-ray changes in OA are:
— joint space narrowing
— subchrondral bony sclerosis
— osteophyte formation
— subchondral cysts
— irregularity of joint surfaces in advanced disease.

Special features in individual joints

HANDS

Heberden's and Bouchard's nodes often show tiny flecks of bone adjacent to the joint line but unattached to the phalanges
In advanced OA deformity of the joint line produces a distinctive 'crinkled smile' appearance.
Erosive changes may be prominent at the DIP and PIP joints in a small percentage of patients; this may give rise to confusion with inflammatory arthritis, particularly psoriatic arthritis.

HIP JOINT

Loss of joint space occurs initially and most prominently at the superior portion of the femoral head adjacent to the acetabulum.

KNEE JOINT

To assess the true degree of joint space narrowing, weight-bearing views should be taken.

DIAGNOSIS

The diagnosis of OA in peripheral joints is usually straightforward.
The most common mistake is to accept radiologically evident OA as the cause of the patient's pain despite features in the history or examination which are inconsistent.
Conversely, the absence of X-ray changes does not exclude OA which may cause severe symptoms early in the disease.

Note:
— atypical distribution suggests secondary OA
— significant stiffness may indicate polymyalgia rheumatica or inflammatory synovitis
— absence of physical signs suggests that pain is not arthritic; neurological or referred pain requires exclusion
— soft tissue lesions particularly enthesopathies, are often confused with osteoarthritis.

MANAGEMENT

Management may include: patient education and reassurance; correction of predisposing or exacerbating factors; drug therapy; local corticosteroid injections; physiotherapy; occupational therapy; the supply of aids and appliances, and surgery.

Patient education

Explanation to the patient should include information about the disease:
— OA is basically due to joint wear and while it is important to preserve muscle power and function, joints should not be overused or excessively strained
— disease progression is usually slow and the extent of involvement remains limited
— function, even in severely affected hands, is generally quite well preserved
— severe disease of the hip or knee, if it should occur, is now amenable to satisfactory surgical correction which preserves mobility.

Correction of predisposing or exacerbating factors

Correctable conditions causing secondary OA should be identified, e.g. unequal leg lengths treated with a shoe raise, repetitive occupational or sporting trauma eliminated.

Obesity, although not proven to cause OA, should be corrected because weight reduction often relieves symptoms in weight-bearing joints and is mandatory if surgery is to be considered.

Depression and systemic illness may reduce well-being, lower the pain threshold and allow attention to be focussed on otherwise mild and well-tolerated OA.

Drug therapy

Drugs do not alter the course of the disease or prevent progression and they have no place in the absence of pain.

DRUGS

Non-steroidal anti-inflammatory drugs (NSAID) are the drugs of choice:
— doses and common side-effects are discussed in Chapter 9
— individual preferences are marked and a 'therapeutic trial' is often necessary.
Analgesics have a limited place.
Other drugs may include antidepressants, mild night sedative.
Systemic corticosteroids and the antirheumatic drugs, gold and D-penicillamine have no place in the management of OA.

Local corticosteroid injections

INDICATIONS

Acute exacerbations or persistent pain and swelling in one or two joints.

CLINICAL USE (*see also* Chapter 9)

Sites of OA particularly suitable for local steroid injections include:
— Bouchard's nodes: inject into the joint capsule *not* the joint line
— carpometacarpal joint of the thumb
— knee joint.

PRECAUTIONS

Never inject a joint or periarticular area if there is any suspicion of local infection.
Injections must always be carried out under aseptic conditions.
Intra-articular injections should not be given into the one joint

too frequently; if there is a need to inject a joint at intervals of less than about 3 months, an alternate solution should be sought to deal with the problem.

Physiotherapy

Therapy includes symptomatic treatment (including packs, short wave diathermy etc.), instruction in exercise, posture, use of walking sticks etc.

Exercises:

1 To restore muscle power and function following orthopaedic surgery. The programme should be devised and supervised by the physiotherapist and the surgeon.

2 For OA of the knee where quadriceps wasting occurs early and allows further joint damage. One of the best active measures for protection and stabilisation of the knee is by developing quadriceps power through correctly performed exercises which limit symptomatic progression of the disease.

Occupational therapy

Occupational therapy contributions include:
— assessment of functional disability
— advice and training in alternate methods of performing various tasks
— instruction in the use of appropriate aids to daily living
— home assessments and the provision of simple modifications such as rails for stairs and beside the bath or toilet, ramps in place of steps and other adjustments which promote the ease and safety of disabled individuals
— design of special splints
— co-ordination of work assessment with government agencies.

Aids and appliances

Aids and appliances fall into several categories which include household and personal aids, shoes, walking aids and splints. Splints may need to be designed for a specific need, e.g. to protect and rest a painful carpometacarpal joint.

Orthopaedic surgery

INDICATIONS

1 Severe pain, inadequately controlled by conservative measures.
2 Marked joint instability or functional impairment, preferably accompanied by significant pain.
3 When these occur in:
— advanced disease
— a joint suitable for surgery
— a patient who wants the operation and has a realistic understanding of what surgery has to offer.

SPECIAL CONSIDERATIONS

Overweight patients, undergoing surgery on lower limb joints, should lose weight.

Peripheral vascular disease may contraindicate surgery on the knee or foot.

Patients should be willing to undertake the necessary post-operative exercise programme; those with OA of the knee benefit from having strong quadriceps muscles prior to operation.

Surgery on one hip or knee is of limited value if other lower limb joints are too damaged to allow improved functions. In such situations, the operation being considered should, by itself, allow significant symptomatic improvement or it must be planned as one of a series of procedures.

OPERATIONS

Basic types of operation involve:
— realignment: osteotomy
— stabilization: arthrodesis
— mobilization: arthroplasty including excision arthroplasty, e.g. Keller's operation, and replacement arthroplasty, e.g. total hip replacement.

Some of the advantages and disadvantages of these procedures are shown in Table 21.1. The decision as to which operation is most suitable for the individual patient involves a variety of technical factors and is made, ultimately, by the orthopaedic surgeon.

New operations and joint prostheses are constantly being

Table 21.1 Comparison of basic surgical procedures

	Osteotomy	Arthrodesis	Total joint arthroplasty
Advantages	Pain relief usually good Joint left intact Further procedures still possible	Pain relief guaranteed Maximum joint stability Long-term result maintained	Pain relief excellent (especially hip) Mobility retained or improved Post-operative recovery quick (3 months) At best, near-normal function
Disadvantages	Joint mobility unimproved Further operations often necessary Post-operative recovery slow Non-union of osteotomy may make later arthroplasty more difficult	Total loss of joint mobility Extra strain on other joints Salvage procedures very difficult Post-operative recovery slow Non-fusion Fusion in malposition	Consistent results for hip; less certain for knee Long-term durability still untested
Complications			Loosening of components Infection of cement/bone interface
Indications	Patients under 50 years Minimal joint destruction Stable joint Applicable to hip and knee	Monoarticular arthritis Useful, for wrist, ankle, tarsus Less ideal for hip and knee	Patients over 50 years or younger patients with built-in physical restraints Ideal for hip Less satisfactory for knee Still experimental for shoulder, elbow and ankle

developed but many years of assessment are necessary before their long-term value can be established.

Joints commonly subjected to surgery of established value include:

Hip. Total hip replacement, when performed skilfully on selected patients, is usually a strikingly successful operation.

Knee.

— osteotomy with or without realignment

— replacement arthroplasty: various types, none yet as regularly satisfactory as total hip replacement.

MTP 1. With hallux valgus or hallux rigidus:

— removal of exostoses and bunion

— Keller's operation, an excision arthroplasty

— arthrodesis of the MTP joint in a slightly extended position.

First carpometacarpal joint (base of the thumb):

— excision arthroplasty

— silastic interposition arthroplasty.

Others. Replacement operations on shoulder or elbow joints are proving successful in some centres.

COURSE AND PROGNOSIS

Once degenerative changes have occurred, they are permanent but the disease, even when slowly progressive, may be asymptomatic. A lack of correlation between radiological changes and symptoms is common in OA involving the hands and first MTP joint.

The course is variable and several patterns are seen:

1 Slow progression.

2 Little or no change over years

— occurs particularly in the hands

— symptoms usually mild or absent, e.g. quiescent Heberden's nodes.

3 Stepwise deterioration with periods of rapid disease progression followed by months or years with little change, followed again by deterioration.

4 Intermittent exacerbations unaccompanied by radiological changes.

Functional impairment relates to the site of involvement:

In the hand: DIP and PIP joint disease, although sometimes causing gross deformity, rarely produces disability comparable to that seen in advanced RA. CMC involvement may be severe and limit the use of the thumb to a marked extent but it is amenable to conservative and surgical management.

At the hip and knee: function may be severely limited but crippling disease resulting in a chair or bedbound existence is now almost restricted to those unfortunate and rare individuals in whom surgery is contraindicated or has failed.

22　Neck and Back Pain

Neck and back pain constitute the biggest problem numerically in most rheumatology practices. In the UK, for example, some 18 million working days are lost each year because of back pain.

While inflammatory diseases, malignant secondaries, infection and metabolic bone disease may all cause spinal pain, in the vast majority of patients, the pain is due to degenerative disease of the disc and vertebral joints, leading to nerve root and sometimes blood vessel entrapment.

Acute cervical disc prominence

Acute cervical prominence usually follows trauma, especially traffic accidents involving 'whiplash' injuries. There is usually a combination of severe neck stiffness and pain, and nerve root irritation, most commonly C5 or C6. The main clinical features of cervical root lesions are summarised in Table 22.1.

Table 22.1　Main features of cervical root lesions.

Root	Sensory symptoms	Motor weakness	Reflex
C2	Occipital pain	—	—
C5	Deltoid region	Shoulder abduction Elbow flexion	Biceps
C6	Thumb and forefinger	Wrist extension	Supinator
C7	Middle finger	Elbow extension	Triceps
C8	Little and ring finger	Flexion of fingers	—

Severe cervical disc protrusion may result in cord compression and require immediate neurosurgery, though the majority of cases improve with immobilisation.

Cervical spondylosis

The majority of people over the age of 50 show radiological evidence of OA of the cervical spine, together with osteophyte formation and disc narrowing (especially C5-6). For this reason, there is frequently a poor correlation between clinical features and radiological change in the cervical spine.

The symptoms are often chronic, recurring and diffuse; as well as neck pain and stiffness, they frequently include pains in one or both shoulders and upper arms, or occipital pains. Associated features may include vertebral ischaemia and brachial neuralgia. The patient may also have the features of lumbar spondylosis, increasing the rheumatic symptoms.

For reasons ill-understood, shoulder rotator cuff syndromes, tennis elbow and medial epicondylitis ('golfer's elbow') are more frequent and recurrent in the presence of cervical spondylosis.

The *physical signs* include limitation of neck movement—flexion, extension, left and right rotation, and left and right lateral flexion—limitation of rotation and lateral flexion are most common, and root signs.

INVESTIGATIONS

Investigations include lateral cervical spine X-rays (largely to exclude other diseases), oblique views if a localised encroachment on one particular nerve root is suspected, as well as routine chest X-ray, full blood count and ESR. One disease which may present diagnostic similarities is polymyalgia rheumatica, with neck and shoulder stiffness, and tenderness over the cervical spine processes, however, the ESR is high.

TREATMENT

In the majority of patients, the symptoms fluctuate and only rarely progress to the stage where surgery is contemplated. A soft flexible collar worn at night often provides relief throughout most of the following day (whether this limits extreme movements of the neck during sleep is uncertain).

Traction or manipulation, provided that neurological features are absent, are popular. While these forms of treatment have rarely been the subject of scientific scrutiny, they provide active therapy and seem to be helpful in the majority of patients.

Acute lumbar disc disease

The onset is often dramatic and spectacular, e.g. the patient is 'paralysed' at an airport whilst picking up a suitcase. As well as severe local back pain, there may be a sensation of 'locking'. Either at the same time, or within hours, there may be sciatic pain which can become the dominant feature. The sciatic and back pain are made worse by all spine and leg movements, as well as by coughing or sneezing.

In the acute stage, there may also be evidence of bladder disturbance.

EXAMINATION

Provided that the pain is not too extreme, limitation of straight leg raising is usual in the presence of disc protrusion. The main features of lumbar root irritation are given in Table 22.2.

Table 22.2   Main features of lumbar root lesions.

Root	Sensory symptoms	Motor weakness	Reflex
L2-4	Front of thigh and knee	Hip flexion Knee extension	Knee jerk
L5	Dorsum of foot Medial side of calf	Dorsiflexion of foot	—
S1	Lateral border of calf and foot Soles	Plantar flexion of foot	Ankle jerk

The commonest discs involved are the two lowest—L4/5 and L5/S1. See Fig. 22.1.

TREATMENT

The majority of patients improve at home with a few days' analgesia and bed rest, preferably on a hard mattress; some patients find relief by sleeping on the floor. Traditionally, severe cases are admitted for 2 weeks' strict bed rest. Leg traction may provide some symptomatic relief, possibly by helping to immobilise the patient.

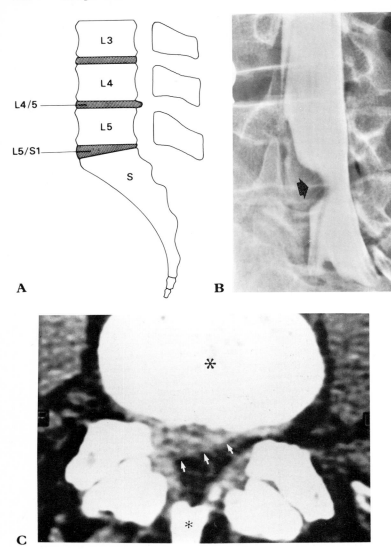

Fig. 22.1 Acute lumbar disc disease. **A** Diagram showing discs involved. **B** Water soluble contrast material in the subarchnoid space outlines the large herniated fragment. **C** Same patient. Herniated lumber or
intervertebral disc. CT scan without contrast material clearly shows the
herniated nucleus pulposus (arrows). Modern CT scanners often show
herniation well enough that myelography is not required. Large asterisk:
vertebral body. Small asterisk: spinous process. (Dr David Lewall, King
Faisal Specialist Hospital, Saudi Arabia.)

Epidural analgesia (infiltration on the extradural space with local anaesthetic) is widely used in the acute stage of the disease, and often provides lasting relief. Surgery is usually reserved for those with serious neurological impairment or the rare case of recurrent or intractable disc disease.

Lumbar spondylosis

As in the case of the cervical spine, X-rays of patients over 40 complaining of low back pain will almost invariably show spondylosis, i.e. one or more areas of disc space narrowing, osteophyte formation, degenerative changes in the posterior joints. Again, the main reason for radiology is in the differential diagnosis of other cases of low back pain such as spondylolisthesis (Fig. 22.2), spondylitis, osteomyelitis, metastases or metabolic bone disease.

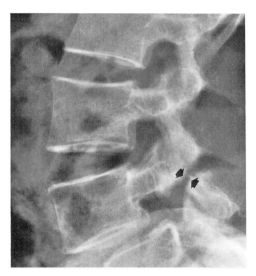

Fig. 22.2   Spondylolisthesis and spondylitis. The pars interarticularis is open (arrows), probably due to a stress fracture. The vertebral body is therefore free to slip forward on the body below (spondylolisthesis). (Dr David Lewall, King Faisal Specialist Hospital, Saudi Arabia.)

SYMPTOMS

Recurrent or chronic low back pain, together with pain referred to one or other leg or gluteal region are the main symptoms.

Occasionally, atypical sciatic pain may present as, for example, calf pain, in the absence of a clear-cut lumbar problem.

SPINAL STENOSIS

Another 'atypical' presentation of lumbar spondylosis is with the constellation of features suggestive of *spinal stenosis*. Usually found in the presence of multiple disc lesions, especially with central disc protrusion, the patient presents with symptoms suggestive of intermittent claudication. On walking, he or she develops pain in one or both thighs or calves.

Characteristically, the pain does *not* come on when the hips are flexed. Thus the patient can cycle on an exercise bicycle for long periods without 'claudication'.

TREATMENT

The high percentage of these patients sitting in rheumatology outpatients, as well as the even higher number attending acupuncture, osteopathy, homeopathy and other non-medical clinics, attests to the inadequacies of treatment. Bedrest and lumbar supports are impractical for the majority of patients. Physiotherapy (including the education of correct back exercises) provides an important part of management. Manipulation (for those with no abnormal neurological signs) is sometimes dramatic in providing short-term relief, and plays an increasing role in management.

Other causes

Other causes of neck and back pain include cancer, Paget's disease (discussed below), Schuermann's syndrome (Fig. 22.3) and TB Brucella (Fig. 22.4).

Paget's disease

Paget's disease is not, strictly speaking, a metabolic bone disease because it is a disorder of individual bones rather than a generalised skeletal abnormality. It is a chronic disease characterised by disorganised osseous architecture with softening, enlargement and weakening of bone.

The aetiology is unkown but some evidence points to the possibility of involvement of a slow virus. Initially there are

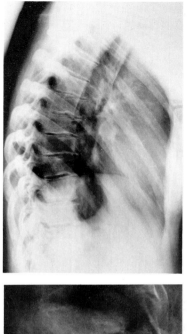

Fig. 22.3   Schuermann's syndrome.

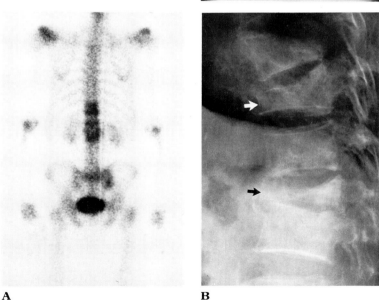

A   **B**

Fig. 22.4   A Brucellosis in a 75 year old Bedoin male. He presented with back pain and undulant fever and admitted drinking fresh camel's milk. The bone scan shows increased uptake at several spinal levels. **B** Lateral view of the spine. Two bodies have become so soft that they have collapsed. The radiological appearance is similar to that of pyogenic osteomyelitis. (Dr David Lewall, King Faisal Specialist Hospital, Saudi Arabia.)

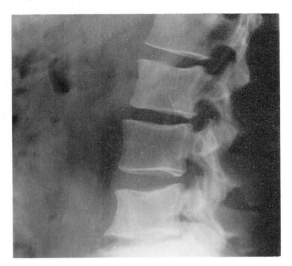

Fig. 22.5   Paget's disease.

increased numbers of large osteoclasts which initiate a lytic phase; this is followed by increased osteoblasts and new bone deposition. Overall bone turnover is increased but the newly formed bone is architecturally chaotic with thickened trabeculae, disorganised osteoid seams and increased vascularity.

The disease occurs in patients over 40 and is more common in males than females. At the age of 50 the prevalence is around 1% but in the very old rises to 10%. Only 5–10% of those affected develop symptoms.

The sites most commonly affected include the pelvis, spine (Fig. 22.5), femur, skull and tibia.

CLINICAL FEATURES

Develop as a result of

Direct bone invovlement
Pain, headache.
Bone deformity and enlargement
— skull enlargement
— kyphosis
— sabre shin
— clavicular and forearm enlargement and bowing fracture.

Bone encroachment causing
Deafness.
Other cranical nerve lesions.
Spinal cord compression.

Effect on joints
Osteoarthritis.

Complications and other features
High output cardiac failure (very rare).
Angioid streaks in the retina.
Hyperuricaemia.
Sarcoma development
— the most serious complication occurring in less than 1% of those affected
— causes increased pain, swelling and usually a rise in alkaline phosphatase.

DIAGNOSIS

Diagnosis is based on
1 The clinical picture.
2 Characteristic biochemistry:
— increased serum alkaline phosphatase
— normal serum calcium and phosphate
— increased urinary hydroxyproline.
3 X-ray showing characteristic features of cortical thickening and a mixed lytic/sclerotic appearance of bone.
4 A bone scan establishing the extent of biopsy.
5 Bone biopsy is rarely necessary.

TREATMENT

Of pagetic bone:
— avoid immobilisation
— calcitonin and disphosphonates.
Of secondary osteoarthritis:
— NSAID
— joint arthroplasty where applicable.

23 Local Rheumatic Disorders

LESIONS OF THE SHOULDER JOINT

Careful examination of the shoulder usually reveals whether the lesion is primarily in the glenohumoral joint or in the periarticular capsular ligaments and tendons. There is frequently accompanying pathology in the cervical spine.

'Frozen' shoulder

All movements are severely limited and painful for a patient suffering from a 'frozen' shoulder. The main features of this serious and disabling condition are:
— older age group
— frequently follows injury to the shoulder
— may follow a hemiplegia or cardiac infarction
— may follow chest surgery
— the pain may continue for weeks or months.

TREATMENT

Treatment consists of analgesia and gentle mobilisation.

Shoulder-hand syndrome

In addition to the 'frozen' shoulder, the hand may become painful and immobile. The skin over the hand becomes puffy and shiny. X-rays may show a patchy or 'spotty' osteoporosis, and joint scans are 'hot'.

The shoulder–hand syndrome, like a 'frozen' shoulder (and other so-called 'reflex' dystrophies or algodystrophies), may follow relatively minor trauma, or alternatively may develop after a cerebrovascular accident or a myocardial infarction.

TREATMENT

Treatments such as sympathectomy, physiotherapy, high dose corticosteroids have all been tried and are rarely obviously successful. In some patients the condition continues for months and years, and depression becomes an important part of the disease.

Supraspinatus tendinitis

The commonest of the 'rotator cuff' lesions, supraspinatus tendinitis involves minor tears or inflammation in the group of muscles and tendons surrounding the glenohumoral joint. There is tenderness laterally over the greater tuberosity, and pain on movement in the characteristic 'painful arc' of 60°–120° as the arm is raised sideways and upwards.

X-rays occasionally reveal opaque deposits of calcium apatite in the region of the supraspinatus tendon (Fig. 23.1).

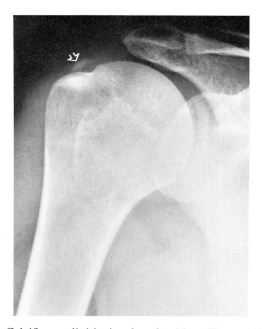

Fig. 23.1 Calcific tendinitis in the shoulder. The calcium deposit (arrow) is in the supraspinatus tendon. When the bicipital tendons are involved the calcium is more difficult to see as it overlies the humeral head. (Dr David Lewall, King Faisal Specialist Hospital, Saudi Arabia.)

TREATMENT

Treatment consists of corticosteroid and local anaesthetic injection into the region of affected tendon.

Bicipital tendonitis

Inflammation of the tendon sheath of the long head of biceps in the bicipital groove frequently accompanies other shoulder lesions. The pain is quite localised, and may be exacerbated when the patient braces the forearm against resistance to flexion.

TREATMENT

Treatment is by local corticosteroid injection.

Subacromial bursitis

Many of the rotator cuff lesions are accompanied by inflammation in the subacromial bursa. Occasionally an effusion may be detected.

TREATMENT

Treatment is by infiltration under the acromion with local anaesthetic and steroids.

The 'Milwaukee' shoulder

A severe form of calcific shoulder disease has been extensively studied by McCarty and colleagues in Milwaukee. It consists of a rotator cuff defect associated with glenohumoral arthritis.

Although rare, it is of interest in that the degenerative shoulder lesion appears to be associated with the presence of large amounts of hydroxyapatite crystals, again providing evidence that some cases of osteoarthritis may have a metabolic or 'crystal-damage' mechanism.

ELBOW LESIONS (Fig. 23.2)

Tennis elbow

Tennis elbow (lateral epicondylitis) results in pain at the tip of the lateral epicondyle, at the attachment of the common extensor muscle origin.

The pain is exacerbated by use of these muscles, e.g. by turning a stiff doorknob.

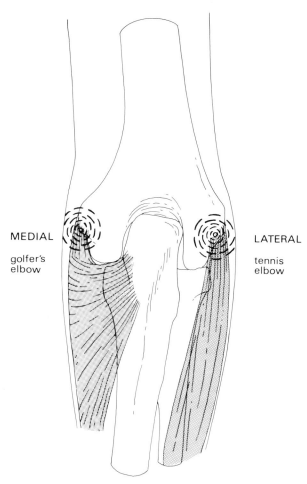

MEDIAL

golfer's
elbow

LATERAL

tennis
elbow

Fig. 23.2   Golfer's and Tennis elbow.

The pain may extend both up and down the arm and, untreated, continue for weeks and months.

TREATMENT

Treatment is by local steroid injection. Re-injection is frequently required. Surgery is needed in very few cases.

Golfer's Elbow (Medial epicondylitis)

Medial epicondylitis, is similar to tennis elbow, though less common. The pain on the tip of the medial epicondyle is usually quite localised.

WRIST LESIONS

Carpal tunnel syndrome (*see* p. 50)

Carpal tunnel syndrome results from compression of the median nerve as it passes under the transverse ligament at the wrist (Fig. 23.3).

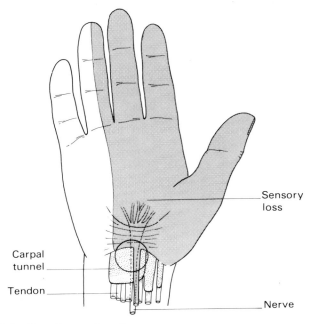

Sensory loss

Carpal tunnel

Tendon

Nerve

Fig. 23.3 Carpal tunnel syndrome

CLINICAL FEATURES

Pain or abnormal sensation in the thumbs, forefinger, middle finger (and medial half of ring finger).
Symptoms common at night.
Tinel's sign—parasthesiae in the above distribution on percussion over the wrist skin creases.
Loss of sensation in the above area.
(Later) weakness and wasting of thenar muscles.

CAUSES

Fluid, e.g. pre-menstrual, post-menopausal.
Synovial swelling, e.g. early RA.
Bone swelling, old injuries etc.
Other, e.g. myxoedema.

TREATMENT

Mild cases—local steroid injection.
Severe cases—surgical decompression.

De Quervain's syndrome

Tenosynovitis of the abductor pollicis longus.
Sometimes associated with swelling over the radial styloid region.
May produce marked disability, e.g. the patient may not be able to hold a cup and saucer or tray.

TREATMENT

Local steroid injection.
Immobilisation and even surgery may be required in resistant cases.

HIP

Trochanteric bursitis

Of the numerous bursae around the hip joint, inflammation in the bursa overlying the greater trochanter may cause considerable pain to the patient and some diagnostic difficulty.

The tenderness is lateral.

Groin pain (characteristic of hip pathology) is absent.

There may be swelling over the lateral aspect of the thigh.

The pain is increased by abduction of the leg against resistance.

TREATMENT

Treatment is by local steroid injection.

FOOT PAIN

In addition to the diseases affecting the various joints of the foot, a number of non-articular causes of foot pain, especially neurological and tendinous may cause acute or chronic foot pain. Both Achilles tendinitis and plantar fasciitis may be traumatic or idiopathic. Plantar fasciitis is an important cause of pain in the heel on walking. Although it is probably most commonly of traumatic origin the relationship to ankylosing spondylitis, Reiter's disease and other seronegative arthropathies has increased awareness that 'idiopathic' plantar fasciitis or achilles tendinitis may in fact represent a *forme fruste* of these diseases.

It is well-known that amongst relatives of patients with ankylosing spondylitis, there exist those whose only medical complaints are of recurrent heel pain, or tibial tuberosity pain, or recurrent mouth ulcers. These examples point to the possibility that a number of cases of 'soft tissue rheumatism' may in fact represent the mildest examples of more well-recognised rheumatological diseases.

24 Arthritis and Infection

VIRAL ARTHRITIS

Viruses which commonly cause arthritis are:
Hepatitis B
Rubella and rubella vaccine
Arboviruses: (arthropod borne)
— Ross River (Australia)
— Chikungunya (Africa, India, SE Asia)
— O'nyong nyong (Africa)
— Sinbis (Africa, SE Asia).
Others which occasionally or rarely cause arthritis are:
Mumps
Varicella
Infectious mononucleosis
Adenovirus type 7
Smallpox and vaccinia.

Pathogenesis

Two mechanisms appear to be involved in pathogenesis:
1 Viral invasion and replication within the synovium, e.g. rubella.
2 An immune complex disease in which the viral antigen in excess causes a serum sickness type reaction, e.g. Hepatitis B.

In some patients and some viral illnesses, it is likely that both mechanisms operate.
Factors governing individual susceptibility to the development of arthritis during viral infection are poorly understood. Arthritis is generally more common in adults than children. There is a large variation in the frequency of arthritis in individual viral infections:
— majority of adults infected with certain arboviruses
— 10-20% of adults infected with Hepatitis B
— 10-20% of women infected with rubella

— <1% of patients infected with mumps, infectious mononucleosis, etc.

Clinical features

CONSTITUTIONAL FEATURES

These include:
— fever, chills, headache, malaise
— myalgia, sore throat, etc.

ARTHRITIS

May be of variable onset, distribution and duration but typically:
— sudden onset
— symmetrical and polyarticular
— small joints of hands and knees affected
— lasts 1–3 weeks.
Tendinitis and periarticular tenderness may be prominent.

RASH

A rash is common, being generally:
— urticaria in Hepatitis B
— morbilliform in rubella
— maculopapular in Arbovirus infection.

OTHER FEATURES

Other features of viral infection:
— lymphadenopathy
— parotitis, orchitis in mumps
— pericarditis in adenovirus type 7
— meningitis in adenovirus and echovirus.

Laboratory findings

HAEMATOLOGY

Hb normal.
WCC normal, reduced or elevated
— relative lymphocytosis.
— ESR normal or elevated.

SEROLOGY

— Rheumatoid factor negative
— may be positive in rubella
— ANA negative.

SYNOVIAL FLUID

WCC elevated 10 000–30 000/mm^3.
Polymorphonuclear leucocyte or monocyte may predominate.
Mononuclear cells predominent in Ross River arthritis.

Treatment

Treatment is symptomatic with aspirin and other non-steroidal anti-inflammatory drugs.

Typical features of common viral arthritides

HEPATITIS B

May cause three rheumatic diseases:
— arthritis, urticaria
— polyarteritis nodosa
— cryoglobulinaemia.
Incubation period can be up to 6 months.
Arthritis:
— occurs in preicteric phase
— sudden onset
— oligo- or polyarthritis especially hands and knees but may be generalised, including cervical spine
— resolves with onset of jaundice usually in 1–3 weeks.
Laboratory tests:
— HBsAg usually present in blood at presentation
— serum C4, C3, CH50 often transiently reduced
— synovial fluid: WCC with polymorphonuclear leucocyte predominance.

RUBELLA AND RUBELLA VACCINE

Incubation period:
— in natural rubella, rash usually precedes arthritis
— after vaccination, arthritis occurs 2–4 weeks later.

Arthralgia may occur without arthritis.

Arthritis:
— sudden onset
— affects especially the knees, hands and wrists
— duration: 1–3 weeks but recurrences of vaccination-associated arthritis occur in up to 30% of patients over periods up to 3 years
— often severe.

Carpal tunnel syndrome is common.

Laboratory tests:
— RF occasionally positive
— serum complement normal.

ARBOVIRUSES

Arbovirus infection is usually by mosquito vector.

Ross River virus
Occurs in Eastern Australia and Fiji.
Affects adults in summer and autumn.

Arthritis:
— sudden onset
— usually polyarticular especially ankles, feet and hands
— usually lasts 2–3 weeks, occasionally months.

Maculopapular rash.

Laboratory tests:
— mononuclear cells predominate in synovial fluid.

BACTERIAL ARTHRITIS

Bacteria are associated with arthritis in several ways:

Septic arthritis The most obvious mechanism is direct invasion of the joint with bacterial multiplication within the articular cavity.

Neisserial arthritis N. gonorrhoeae and N. meningitidis may cause a bacteraemia followed by septic arthritis; in addition, they cause an aseptic arthritis apparently mediated by an immune response to the Neisserial infection with formation of immune complexes. (*See* p. 257).

Reactive or post-infective arthritis Some infections are followed by arthritis which is invariably sterile. These have been called reactive or post-infective arthritis and include rheumatic fever and arthritis following sexually acquired and enteric infections (including Reiter's syndrome). See Chapter 25.

SEPTIC ARTHRITIS

Bacteria most likely to cause septic arthritis at different ages and in specially predisposed individuals are shown in Table 24.1.

Table 24.1   Bacteria likely to cause septic arthritis

Patient	Organism
Child	
Neonate	*S. aureus*
	E. coli
Age 1 month–2 years	*H. influenzae*
	S. aureus
Age 2 years +	*S. aureus*
	Various enteric organisms
	H. influenzae
Adult	
Healthy	*N. gonococcus*
	S. aureus
RA	*S. aureus*
Alcohol and drug abuse	*S. pneumoniae*
	Various enteric organisers
	Pseudomonas, Serratia

These particularly include:
Staphlococcus aureus
Neisseria gonorrhoeae
Haemophilus influenzae
Streptococcus pyogenes
Escherichia coli and other Gram negative organisms.

Pathogenesis

It is most unusual to see septic arthritis in an otherwise healthy adult with normal joints.

PREDISPOSING FACTORS

Local:
— joint damaged by RA, OA, etc.
— presence of joint prosthesis.

Systemic:
— immunosuppressed patient
  steroids, cytotoxic drugs
  malignancy
  uraemia
— diabetes
— sickle cell disease
— alcoholism
— splenectomy
— i.v. drug abuse.

Organism entry may follow:
— haematogenous spread from site of infection
— direct spread, e.g. from osteomyelitis or local infection
— inoculation, e.g. contaminated intra-articular injection.

JOINT DAMAGE

Proteolytic and lysosomal enzymes released by polymorphonuclear leucocytes rapidly damage proteoglycans.

Irreversible damage follows disruption of the collagen network and chondrocyte death.

Clinical features

TYPICAL PRESENTATION

Typical presentation is a febrile, toxic patient suffering from a 'hot, red joint' with:
— monoarticular involvement, commonly the knee, usually a large joint but any joint may be affected
— exquisitely tender
— movement producing severe pain.

ATYPICAL PRESENTATION

Patients who are very young, old, sick, immunosuppressed or have RA, i.e. those most at risk of developing septic arthritis, often show an atypical clinical picture.
Constitutional features may be inconspicuous:
— mild anorexia
— occasional chills
— low grade fever.
Joint involvement may be oligoarticular or even polyarticular.
Joints may be warm, only slightly tender and show a relatively good range of movement.
In the patient with RA and infection, one joint may become slightly more painful, warm and tender and is often mistaken for a flare of the rheumatoid synovitis.

Laboratory findings

HAEMATOLOGY

Leucocytosis:
— present in 50–70% of patients, i.e. absent in 30–50%, so *not* a reliable guide at presentation.
ESR typically elevated.

SYNOVIAL FLUID

Purulent: WCC usually $>50\,000/cm$, $>90\%$ polymophonuclear leucocytes.
Low glucose.
Gram stain and/or culture:
— positive in 50–70%
— usually negative if antibiotics already given.

CULTURES

Other cultures may be positive, e.g. blood, urine, sputum, skin lesions, genital, nasopharynx.

RADIOLOGY

X-rays should be obtained to establish baseline, but if early in course, they show:
— soft tissue swelling
— later, osteoporosis.
After 10–14 days, changes may include:
— joint space narrowing
— periarticular bone lysis
— joint destruction (Fig. 24.1) and disorganisation.

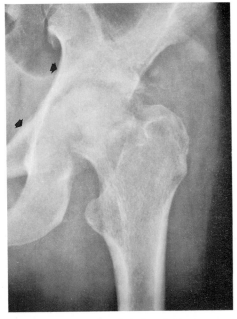

Fig. 24.1 Septic Hip. This rather indolent infection started in the joint and has destroyed cartilage and bone. The destructive process has extended through the acetabulum to stimulate new bone formation along the pelvic brim (arrows). Tuberculosis can have an identical appearance. (Dr David Lewall, King Faisal Specialist Hospital, Saudi Arabia.)

Diagnosis and differential diagnosis

Diagnosis is based on suspicion:
— typical clinical picture
— possible sepsis in susceptible patient.

Confirmation is by demonstration of organisms in a joint on Gram stain or culture of synovial fluid.

Differential diagnosis:

'Hot red joint', i.e. acute monoarthritis:
— infection
— crystal synovitis—gout, pseudogout
— acute haemarthrosis
— acute seronegative arthritis—rarely, e.g. Reiter's syndrome, psoriatic arthritis.

Acute polyarthritis:
— infection
— post-infective arthritis
— rheumatic fever
— serum sickness
— viral arthritis.

Management

If septic arthritis is suspected, the following steps are essential:
1 Obtain synovial fluid *immediately*.
2 Obtain other specimens for culture:
— blood
— any skin lesion
— nasopharyngeal
— genital, rectal
— other: urine, sputum, stool, etc.
3 Commence parenteral antibiotics. Choice of antibiotic will be determined by synovial fluid Gram stain result or most likely organism based on patient's age, clinical condition, etc. (*see* Table 23.1) and/or subsequently on synovial fluid culture and antibiotic sensitivity results.

Duration of antibiotic therapy is influenced by various factors: parenteral antibiotics are usually continued for 2–4 weeks with oral antibiotics for a further 4 weeks.

For gonococcal infections, 2 weeks antibiotic therapy is usually considered adequate.

No advantage has been demonstrated from the use of intra-articular antibiotics which may induce a chemical synovitis.
4 Immobilise joint—splint in a position of function. Remobilis-ation with passive and later active exercises may commence once pain is settled.
5 Orthopaedic surgical consultation.

6 Joint drainage. Needle drainage under local anaesthetic with a wide bore needle is usually adequate. This should be repeated daily while a purulent effusion persists.

Indication for surgical drainage include:
— persistent febrile course
— thick pus
— inaccessible joint, e.g. sacroiliac joint.

NEISSERIAL ARTHRITIS

Arthritis associated with neisserial infections is now a major world wide disease.

Gonococcal infection

Arthritis complicates gonococcal infection in 1–3% of patients.

CLINICAL FEATURES

Clinical features of disseminated gonococcal infection:
— most common in young people (age < 40) with a predominance of females
— onset is commonly within one week of menstruation or during pregnancy (always obtain a detailed menstrual history)
— common in homosexuals.

Systemic features may be prominent:
— fever, rigors
— leucocytosis.

Arthritis:
— migratory polyarthritis which may localise to oligoarthritis or monoarthritis
— tenosynovitis is common especially around the wrists, hands and ankles.

Skin lesions are characteristic but usually sparse:
— a tender, pustular or necrotic lesion on an erythematous base due to vasculitis
— Gram stain in culture of fresh lesion may show gonococci.

Other metastatic sepsis may occur as a result of bacteraemia, e.g. endocarditis or meningitis.

DIAGNOSIS

A diagnosis is suspected on the basis of the characteristic clinical picture in a susceptible individual.

Synovial fluid is typically unhelpful, and usually inflammatory with WCC >40 000/cm; >90% polymorphonuclear leucocytes, but culture is positive in <50%.
Gram stain may show G-ve intracellular diplococci in specimens from the urethra, fresh skin lesions or synovial fluid.
Positive cultures may be obtained from blood, cervix, urethra, rectum, pharynx or synovial fluid.

TREATMENT

Penicillin is the antibiotic of choice although some examples of arthritis due to penicillin resistant gonococcus have been reported.
Therapeutic response usually occurs within a few days.
Short-term antibiotic therapy is effective: 2 weeks' treatment is generally sufficient.
Septic arthritis is treated as outlined in the preceding section.

Meningococcal infection

Arthritis complicates meningococcal infection in 2–10% of patients.
Septic arthritis may occur but an aseptic reactive arthritis is more usual; there is some evidence that a hypersensitivity reaction, mediated by immune complexes containing meningococcal antigen, play a role in the aseptic arthritis.

CLINICAL FEATURES

Arthritis occurs after the other manifestations of meningococcaemia and its onset is unaffected by the use or efficacy of antibiotics.
Usually oligoarticular, sometimes polyarticular.
Skin lesions, like those of disseminated gonococcal infection may occur.
Tenosynovitis is unusual.

TREATMENT

Septic arthritis: treatment according to the principles outlined previously with high dose penicillin.
Aseptic arthritis:
— treatment of meningococcaemia is continued with penicillin

— arthritis is treated symptomatically with non-steroidal anti-inflammatory drugs and rest.

MYCOBACTERIAL INFECTIONS

Tuberculosis

Tuberculosis may primarily affect either bone or synovium or spread to one site from the other.

PATHOGENESIS AND PATHOLOGY

Of tuberculous infections, about 1% of patients have osteomyelitis or synovitis.
Up to 50% have coexistent pulmonary tuberculosis.
Skeletal infection follows:
— haematogenous spread
— lymphatic spread from local lesions
— reactivation.
Sites affected:
— spine 50%
— large weight-bearing joints 30–40%.
Infection provokes granulomatous response; destructive changes usually occur slowly. In articular disease, subchondral bone erosions often precede cartilagenous destruction with relative preservation of joint space until the disease is well advanced.

COMMON PRESENTATIONS

Common presentations are:
— spondylitis
— chronic monoarthritis.

SPINAL TUBERCULOSIS

Sites of spinal tuberculosis include:
— thoracic and lumbar spine more commonly affected than cervical
— multiple sites may be involved and skip lesions may occur following haematogenous spread
— sacroiliac joints usually unilaterally involved.

Clinical features
Back pain, tenderness.
Kyphosis.
Nerve root lesions.
Cord compression.
Cold abscess.

PERIPHERAL TUBERCULOSIS

Sites of peripheral tuberculosis:
— hips, knees, ankles, wrists, occasionally fingers
  in joints or surrounding bones.

Clinical features
Low grade inflammatory arthritis:
— pain, swelling, limitation and warmth
— muscle wasting
— cold abscess development.

SYNOVIAL FLUID

Smear for AFB, positive in only about 20%.
Culture for AFB, positive in about 80%.
High protein, often low glucose.
WCC variable, 10 000–20 000/mm^3.

DIAGNOSIS

Skin tests
  Usually positive except in the old or anergic.

Biopsy
Biopsy is the most useful diagnostic procedure:
— histology may show granulomata and stain for AFB
— culture of tissue is positive in about 90%.

Radiology
Spine:
— typically shows vertebral collapse with disc space narrowing
  and paraspinal soft tissue shadow due to abscess formation
  (Fig. 24.2).
Peripheral joints:
— destructive changes are accompanied by little reactive bone
  formation

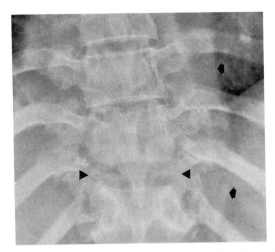

Fig. 24.2A Tuberculosis of the lower thoracic spine. Note the swelling of the paraspinal tissues (arrows). One vertebral body is almost completely destroyed (arrow heads), and the body above has lost its sharp outline due to invasion by the bacilli. (Dr David Lewall, King Faisal Specialist Hospital, Saudi Arabia.)

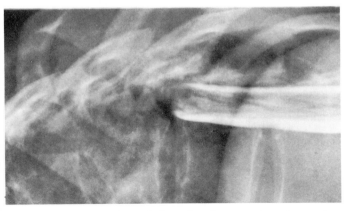

Fig. 24.2B Myelogram, lateral view, showing complete obstruction.

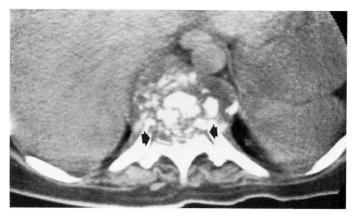

Fig. 24.2C CT scan shows fragmentation of the vertebral body and encroachment into the canal by granulation tissue and bony debris (arrow). This accounts for the obstruction seen on the myelogram. (Dr David Lewell, King Faisal Specialist Hospital, Saudi Arabia.)

— subchondral erosions are common
— joint space may be relatively preserved until there is extensive destruction of adjacent cortical bone
— total joint destruction occurs later (Fig. 24.3).

TREATMENT

Antituberculous drug therapy should be continued for 18–24 months:
Surgery generally reserved for:
— drainage of abscess
— fusion of unstable spine
— arthrodesis of severely damaged joints.

Atypical mycobacteria

Skeletal infection with atypical mycobacteria is rare but they may cause:
— osteomyelitis
— arthritis
— periarthritis
— tenosynovitis.
Diagnosis is usually made on culture of biopsy material.

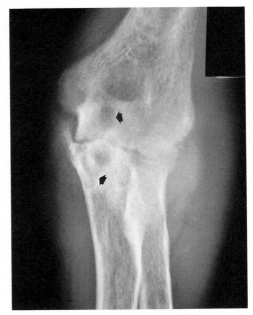

Fig. 24.3 Tuberculous arthritis of the elbow. This is an advanced lesion with destruction of the articular cartilage and invasion of the adjacent bone (arrows). The fate of such lesions is to develop bony ankylosis. (Dr David Lewall, King Faisal Specialist Hospital, Saudi Arabia.)

TREATMENT

Antituberculous drugs: the atypical mycobacteria are relatively resistant to these agents.
Surgery is often indicated to remove infected tissue.

Mycobacterium leprae

Mycobacterium leprae may cause:
— osteomyelitis of phalanges
— Charcot joints due to neuropathy
— arthritis during erythema nodusum leprosum.

SPIROCHAETAL INFECTION

Lyme Disease

Lyme arthritis
Occurs in Eastern USA.

Tick-transmitted disorder, due to a spirochaete.
Arthritis:
— sudden onset
— mono- or oligoarticular involvement of large joints, especially the knee
— often recurrent.
Skin rash: erythema chronicum migrans
— characteristic large red macular or papular rash with central clearing.
Neurological abnormalities may include:
— cranial nerve palsy
— meningitis
— sensory radiculopathy.
Myocardial abnormalities may include AV block.

FUNGAL INFECTION

Fungal infection is a rare cause of skeletal disease but should be considered in:
— unusual arthritis unresponsive to treatment
and
— immunosuppressed individuals.
Generally:
— osteomyelitis is more common than arthritis
— multiple sites may be involved
— X-ray may show lytic and sclerotic lesions
— diagnosis is made on culture of biopsy material.
Fungal diseases which may cause skeletal infection include:
— Candidiasis
— Sporotrichosis
— Aspergillosis
— Histoplasmosis
— Cryptococcosis
— Coccidioidomycosis
— Blastomycosis.
Fungus-like diseases which may cause skeletal infection include:
— Nocardiosis
— Actinomycosis.

25 Reactive Arthritis

The term reactive arthritis refers to arthritis following an identifiable infection in which the causative micro-organism cannot be isolated from the joint. Although, by definition, this term may include certain viral infections, patients with gonococcal arthritis and those with the arthritis of erythema nodosum following infection, recent convention generally restricts its application to two main groups:
— rheumatic fever
— arthritis following sexually acquired and enteric infections.

RHEUMATIC FEVER

Rheumatic fever is an acute inflammatory disease which affects the joints, heart, skin and sometimes the central nervous system as an indirect result of a Group A streptococcal throat infection.

Epidemiology

Age Any age except infancy. Typically affects school age child 5–15 years with peak incidence at about 8 years.

Sex The male to female ratio is equal.

Prevalence Variable. Still a common disease in poorer communities and developing countries.
Rare in industrialised countries with a dramatic decline in incidence incompletely explained by:
— improved socio-economic factors, e.g. sanitation, overcrowding, etc.
— availability of antibiotics.

Aetiology

Rheumatic fever is precipitated by pharyngeal infection with Group A streptococcus.

Prevention of streptococcal throat infection prevents rheumatic fever.

Factors relating to the infection:
Site of infection is important
— pharangeal infection apparently critical.
Streptococcal skin infections may precipitate acute glomerulonephritis but not rheumatic fever.
Group A streptococcus of certain M protein serotypes are more arthritogenic than others.

Factors relating to the host:
Genetic factors
— familial occurrence is common
— concordance in monozygous twins is only about 20%
— no HLA A or B associations although there may be an association with certain B cell allo-antigens.
Socio-economic
— overcrowding correlates strongly with the incidence of rheumatic fever, presumably because it increases the likelihood of contracting streptococcal infection.
Sex and age
— disease does not begin in infancy and first attacks decline sharply during adult life
— chorea does not occur in sexually mature males; arthritis more common with increasing age.

Pathogenesis

The mechanism by which streptococcal pharyngitis causes or triggers rheumatic fever is unknown.
Although:
— cross reactivity has been demonstrated between various streptococcal antigens and human tissues, including heart muscle
— auto-antibodies to heart muscle, particularly sarcolemma membrane, have been found in rheumatic fever
— both humoral and cellular immune response to streptococcal antigens are greater in rheumatic fever patients than in nonrheumatic fever convalescents of streptococcal pharyngitis
— streptococcal toxins can cause direct tissue damage.
None of the theories of pathogenesis incoporating these findings has been validated.

Clinical manifestations

THROAT INFECTION

Up to one-third of patients do not recall pharyngitis.
Sore throat is commonly mild.

LATENT PERIOD

Time between onset of pharyngitis and onset of rheumatic fever:
— range: 1–5 weeks
— average 18 days.
Latent period does not become shorter in recurrent attacks.

ARTHRITIS

Common especially with increasing age.
Occurs early.
Typically:
Very painful with tenderness and limitation of movement although swelling, redness and heat may be inconspicuous.
Large joints affected more than small joints.
Migratory
— several joints affected successively
— persists in any one joint for a few days, rarely for more than one week.
Settles within about 4 weeks.
Chronic changes are absent.
Note:
Arthritis rarely affects the spine, temporomandibular joints or the small joints of the hands or feet.

CARDITIS

Common in children but less frequent with increasing age.
Manisfestations:
— endocarditis: causing valvular lesions
and/or
— myocarditis: causing tachycardia, cardiomegaly, CCF
and/or
— pericarditis.

Note:
Prolonged PR interval (first degree heart block) is common but does not necessarily indicate carditis.

ERYTHEMA MARGINATUM

Uncommon.
Usually occurs early but can persist for months in the absence of other evidence of activity.
Characteristics:
— individual lesions, which may be multiple, begin as an area of erythema which enlarges with a defined pink or red edge and a clearing centre
— may move and change rapidly like 'smoke rings'
— occurs on the trunk and proximal extremities
— not painful or itchy.

SUBCUTANEOUS NODULES

Occur later in course, especially associated with cardiac involvement.
Round, firm, painless, mobile subcutaneous lesions up to 2 cm diameter.
Occur in crops over tendons and bony prominences: scalp, occiput, extensor tendons of hands, feet, elbows, knees, vertebral spine, Achilles tendon.
Lasts days to weeks.

CHOREA (SYDENHAM'S CHOREA, ST VITUS DANCE)

May be the sole manifestation of rheumatic fever.
Rarely occurs at the same time as arthritis.
More common in girls and does not affect sexually mature males.
May follow streptococcal infection with a latent period of 1–6 months.
Lasts 1 week to 2 years, usually 2–3 months.
Manifestations:
— involuntary, rapid purposeless movements—affecting face, hands, feet, speech, causing marked clumsiness, difficulty with handwriting, etc.—which disappears during sleep
— muscular weakness
— emotional lability.

On follow-up studies, up to 20% of patients with chorea as the only apparent manifestation of rheumatic fever have evidence of heart disease (Note: some cases may have been SLE).

OTHER FEATURES

Fever occurs at onset: often persistent, 38–40°C, rarely lasts for more than 4 weeks.
Abdominal pains.
Epistaxis.

Recurrences

Common; occur only after a further streptococcal infection.
Most common following infection which produces a marked serological response.
Occur particularly in young patients, usually within several years of the first attack and in patients with carditis.
Although manifestations typically repeat those of the initial attack, the prevalence of heart disease increases with the number of attacks.

Laboratory tests

FOR STREPTOCOCCAL INFECTION

Supporting previous streptococcal infection
1 Serological:
— except in those with chorea as the sole manifestation of rheumatic fever, patients invariably show serological evidence of recent streptococcal infection.
Streptococcal antibody tests:
— anti-streptolysin 0 titre (ASOT): 80% positive at onset
— anti-DNAase B   ⎫
— anti-hyaluronidase   ⎬   one positive in the remaining 20%
— anti-streptokinase   ⎭
Streptozyme test. Detects antibodies to:
— mixture of streptococcal antigens
— simple, quick and very sensitive
— positive in 100% of cases of rheumatic fever.
2 Culture of throat swab:
— often negative by time of onset of rheumatic fever.

FOR SYSTEMIC INFLAMMATION

Supporting systemic inflammation:
— ESR elevated
— C reaction protein elevated
— leucocytosis; normochromic normocytic anaemia
— other acute phase reactants elevated
    α_2 and γ globulin
    complement

OTHER TESTS

ANA and rheumatoid factor negative.
Other tests of joint and heart involvement:
— ECG: conduction disturbances
— chest X-ray may show cardiomegaly.
Synovial fluid analysis
— sterile
— inflammatory: WCC 1000–80 000/mm³ predominantly polymorphonuclear leucocytes.

Diagnosis

MODIFIED JONES CRITERIA

1 *Major Manifestations*:
Carditis
Polyarthritis
Chorea
Erythema marginatum
Subcutaneous nodules
2 *Minor Manifestations*:
Clinical
— fever
— arthralgia
— previous rheumatic fever or rheumatic heart disease.
Laboratory
— elevated ESR or CRP
— leucocytosis
— prolonged PR interval.
3 *Other features:*
Supporting evidence of preceding streptococcal infection
— increase in ASOT or other streptococcal antibody

— positive throat cultures
— recent scarlet fever.

Diagnosis of rheumatic fever highly probable with
— two major criteria   ⎫ If supported by evidence of
— one major and two minor   ⎬ preceding streptococcal
  criteria   ⎭ infection
Note:
The terms 'major' and 'minor' manifestations refer to their diagnostic significance not to their frequency or clinical importance.

DIFFERENTIAL DIAGNOSIS

Differential diagnosis of fever and polyarthritis:
1   Systemic onset JCA (Still's disease):
— fever is typically remittant
— infants may be affected
— arthritis involving small joints of hands, feet and cervical spine common
— rash is evanescent but macular.
Note:
ASOT often elevated in Still's disease.
2   SBE:
— especially in patients with rheumatic heart disease
— may present as polyarthritis following throat infection
— blood cultures essential to differentiate febrile patients with murmur and arthritis.
3   Gonococcal polyarthritis:
— especially in adolescents and young adults.
4   Serum sickness:
— may follow antibiotic treatment of throat infection
— urticaria and lymphadenopathy are common.
5   Viral infections:
— especially Hepatitis B, rubella, etc.
6   SLE:
— ANA and other serology usually positive.
— CRP low in SLE.
7   Other forms of reactive arthritis.
8   Sickle cell anaemia.
Differential diagnosis of chorea:
1   Ticks.
2   SLE.

Treatment

Establish diagnosis.
Bed rest for first 3 weeks.
Regular clinical assessment for the development of carditis.
Eradicate streptococcal infection and establish prophylactic regimen.
Aspirin (60–90 mg/kg/day) is used to treat
— fever
— arthritis
— carditis without CCF.
Corticosteroids: although there is no clear evidence that they reduce residual rheumatic heart disease, they are used to treat
— severe carditis especially with CCF
— fever, severe arthritis, etc. uncontrolled by high dose salicylates.

Carditis
Diuretics may be required.
Digoxin readily causes toxicity in rheumatic carditis and must be used with caution.

Chorea
Tranquillisers such as diazepam may be needed.

DURATION OF TREATMENT

Usually continued for 4 weeks and if the patient clinically satisfactory, it is tapered over the next 2 weeks.
'Rebound' does not occur if the disease has been quiescent for more than 2 months after the discontinuation of salicylates or steroids.

Prevention of recurrence

Prophylactic antibiotic treatment can effectively prevent recurrences of rheumatic fever.
Most effective regimen:
— 1.2 million units benzathine penicillin G im injection every 4 weeks.
Less effective alternative oral regimens:
— oral penicillin V 125–250 mg bd
— erythromycin 250 mg bd.

ARTHRITIS FOLLOWING INFECTION

Reactive arthritis following sexually acquired and enteric infection is relatively uncommon but it is an important example of the interaction between genetic predisposition and environmental factors in the production of inflammatory arthritis. The concept of reactive arthritis is an evolving one and is characterised by three notable features.

1   The same clinical entity may be triggered by various infective precipitants.

Reiter's syndrome is a form of reactive arthritis which may occur following sexually acquired urethritis. However, the same syndrome may occur after a variety of enteric infections and occasionally in the absence of any obvious infective event.

2   The same triggering infection may precipitate various clinical entities. Sexually acquired non-specific urethritis and various enteric infections may precipitate a spectrum of clinical entities ranging from arthritis alone, through various 'incomplete' forms of Reiter's syndrome to the full Reiter's combination of arthritis, urethritis, conjunctivitis, uveitis and mucocutaneous lesions.

3   These entities all show a common genetic predisposition.

HLA-B27 is present in 40–70% of patients with either sexually acquired reactive arthritis, arthritis associated with enteric infections or typical Reiter's syndrome.

Thus, reactive arthritis must be regarded as a spectrum of entities triggered by various infective agents in patients with a common genetic predisposition.

Infective agents

Identified infective agents which can precipitate these types of arthritis include:
Sexually acquired infections:
— Chlamydia trachomatis
— Ureaplasma.
Enteric infections:
— Shigella flexneri
— Salmonella
— Yersinia enterocolitica
— Clostridium difficile
— Campylobacter.

Others:
— ? streptococci.

LATENT PERIOD

Latent period usually 1–3 weeks after infection.

CLINICAL MANIFESTATIONS

(*See also* Reiter's syndrome, Chap. 10.)

Arthritis
Typically asymmetrical and oligoarthritis:
— but may be monoarticular or polyarticular
— predominantly lower limbs—knees and ankles.
Sausage toes:
— diffuse swelling of a whole toe due to a combination of teno-synovitis and small joint synovitis.
Low back pain and radiological sacroiliitis may occur.
Usually settles within about 3 months but occasionally protracted enthesopathy may occur.
Other features include:
— conjunctivitis, uveitis
— mucocutaneous lesions.

TREATMENT

Treatment of infection does not influence course of arthritis.
Treatment of arthritis:
— physical measures
— non-steroidal anti-inflammatory drugs: indomethacin, phenyl-butazone
— local steroid injections.

26 Arthritis in Systemic Disease

Rheumatic symptoms feature prominently in the presentation or course of a great number of systemic diseases. This highlights the need to assess rheumatological complaints in the light of the general medical condition and past history and to avoid assuming too readily that aches, pains, arthralgia and even arthritis are due to a rheumatic disease.

CARDIOVASCULAR DISEASES

Congenital cyanotic heart disease

Congenital cyanotic heart disease may be complicated by:
— hyperuricaemia and gout, secondary to polycythaemia
— hypertrophic osteoarthropathy.

Bacterial endocarditis

Manifestations may include:
— arthralgia and arthritis: oligo- or monoarticular, and poly-arthritis (possibly immune-complex)
— hypertrophic osteoarthropathy.
Note:
Rheumatoid factor is positive in up to 50% of patients with bacterial endocarditis.

Ischaemic heart disease

The commonly observed clustering of obesity, ischaemic heart disease, hypertension and hyperlipidaemia commonly includes hyperuricaemia and sometimes gout.

ENDOCRINE DISEASES

Acromegaly

The effect of excessive growth hormone on connective tissues can result in a number of musculoskeletal problems:
— carpal tunnel syndrome
— proximal myopathy
— back pain (probably related to hypermobility and accelerated spondylosis)
— peripheral arthritis.

Peripheral arthritis is a degenerative arthropathy distinguished from primary osteoarthritis by:
— hypermobility, especially early
— distribution, commonly polyarticular, affecting wrists, MCP and other large and small joints

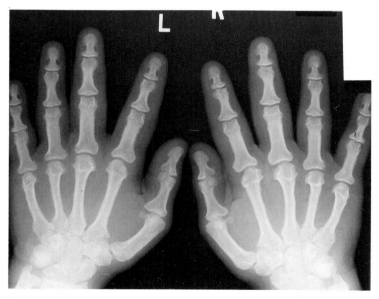

Fig. 26.1 Acromegaly (hands).

— X-rays show osteophytes with increased joint space (Fig. 26.1). A useful radiological sign is increased thickness of the heel pad (Fig. 26.2).

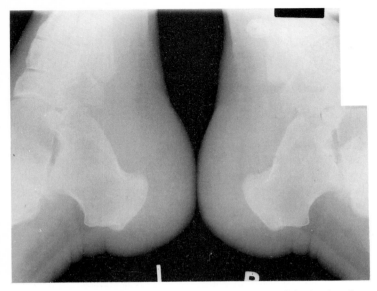

Fig. 26.2   Acromegaly (heel) – increased thickening of the heel pad.

Hypothyroidism

Rheumatic manifestations are common in primary hypothyroidism:
— carpel tunnel syndrome
— proximal myopathy (aches, pains and muscular stiffness; proximal weakness is not usually prominent)
— arthropathies (non-inflammatory effusions; calcium pyrophosphate deposition).

Hyperthyroidism

Myopathy with proximal weakness is the main feature with hyperthyroidism.
Thyroid acropachy:
— a rare complication of Graves' disease
— resembles hypertrophic pulmonary osteoarthropathy and is characterised by clubbing of fingers and toes, periostitis of distal extremities and digits, and thickening of soft tissues of fingers.

Hyperparathyroidism

With its profound effects on bone, muscles and calcium metabolism and its complex relationship with renal function, parathyroid hormone excess may cause a wide variety of musculoskeletal manifestations.

Parathyroid bone disease
A generalised bone disorder due to the resorptive effects of parathyroid hormone and characterised by:
— osteoporosis with vertebral collapse and other fractures following slight trauma
— single or multiple bone cysts with osteitis fibrosa cystica (Fig. 26.3)
— subperiosteal resorption of bone (Fig. 26.4) seen particularly along radial borders of middle phalanges and outer third of clavicle
— 'ground glass' appearance of skull.

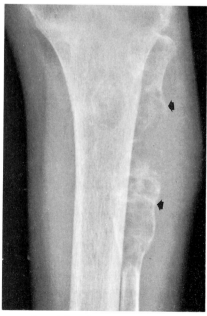

Fig. 26.3   Hyperparathyroidism is a 26 year old woman. There is a large brown tumour in the fibula (arrows). These occur mainly in the primary form of this disease. (Dr David Lewall, King Faisal Specialist Hospital, Saudi Arabia.)

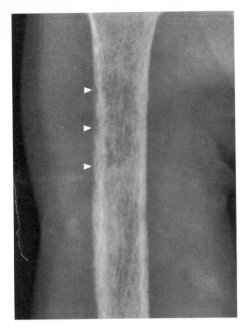

Fig. 26.4 Superiosteal bone resorption in the humerus. Resorption imparts a lacey appearance to the cortex (arrow heads). It is usually best seen on the radial side of the phlanges and is the most useful radiologic sign of hyperparathyroidism. (Dr David Lewall, King Faisal Specialist Hospital, Saudi Arabia.)

Rheumatoid like erosive arthritis
— symmetrical inflammatory polyarthritis affecting particularly hands, wrists and feet
— X-rays show juxta-articular erosions like rheumatoid arthritis which occur with or without subperiosteal resorption.

Ankylosing spondylitis-like spinal changes
— back pain and stiffness with thoracic kyphosis and loss of lumbar lordosis
— X-rays show sacroiliac erosions or fusion and paravertebral calcification.

Chondrocalcinosis
— occurs in up to 25% of patients
— occasional attacks of pseudogout.

Gout
— hyperuricaemia is due to renal tubular defect.

Extra-articular calcification:
— ectopic calcification occurs in hyperparathyroidism secondary to renal insufficiency
— may cause inflammatory periarthritis.

Myopathy
— generalised muscle weakness may be a presenting feature.

Hypoparathyroidism

Ankylosing spondylitis-like spinal changes:
— pain, stiffness and limitation of spine
— X-rays may show paraspinal calcification with sacroiliac joints usually normal.

Acute pseudogout
— may follow parathyroidectomy.

Diabetes

Diabetes is a common disorder and a number of rheumatic diseases have been reported in association with it although in many instances, the true extent of the association is uncertain.

Neuropathic arthropathy
— results from neuropathy
— usually involves the forefoot, especially MTP and interphalangeal joints.

Osteolysis of distal foot
— reported in the absence of significant neurological or vascular pathology.

Soft tissue lesions with increased prevalence of
— Dupuytren's contractures
— shoulder capsulitis
— flexion contraction of fingers in juvenile onset diabetes.

Associations of uncertain validity
— hyperuricaemia and gout
— calcium pyrophosphate deposition
— senile ankylosing vertebral hyperostosis.

GASTROENTEROLOGICAL DISEASES

Inflammatory bowel disease (*see* Chap. 10)

Ulcerative colitis.
Crohn's disease—regional enteritis.

Whipple's disease

Whipple's disease is rare, occurring predominantly in men and characterised by:
— diarrhoea
— fevers
— pigmentation
— lymphadenopathy
— arthritis.
It is apparently due to infection:
— PAS staining granules found in macrophages in interstitial mucosa, synovium and lymph nodes
— rod-shaped organism identified in intestinal mucosa on electron microscopy
— although never transmitted and no organisms cultured, PAS positive granules disappear after antibiotic treatment.

Intestinal Bypass

Intestinal bypass surgery, performed for gross obesity, is complicated by polyarthritis and/or tenosynovitis in 30% of patients following jejunocolostomy and 10% of patients following jejunoileostomy.
Synovitis presumed due to sensitivity reaction to bacteria colonising the blind loop.
Restoration of bowel continuity cures the arthritis.

Pancreatic Disease

Acute pancreatitis and pancreatic carcinoma may be complicated by:
— nodular subcutaneous fat necrosis
— acute arthritis especially of knees and ankles.

Liver Disease

Common manifestations of active chronic hepatitis include:
— arthralgia and arthritis
— SLE-like syndrome
— Sjogren's syndrome.
Primary biliary cirrhosis may occur in association with CREST syndrome.

HAEMOPOIETIC DISEASES

Haemophilia

Factor VIII deficiency and other bleeding disorders may cause two types of joint problem: acute haemarthrosis and chronic arthropathy.

ACUTE HAEMARTHROSIS

Onset usually in childhood.
Trauma often mild or absent.
Usually monoarticular.
Affects particularly the knee (Fig. 26.5), elbow or ankle.

Clinical Features:
Rapid onset.
Very painful, tender, hot, red joint.
Markedly limited by pain.

Differential diagnosis
Differential diagnosis is septic arthritis.

Treatment
Replacement of deficient clotting factor as soon as possible.
Temporary joint immobilisation.
Symptomatic treatment with analgesics, ice packs.
Joint aspiration if effusion very tense.
Active remobilisation as soon as acute phase has settled.
Treated correctly, initial episode resolves completely.

CHRONIC ARTHROPATHY

Chronic arthropathy is a characteristic degenerative arthropathy followed by recurrent haemarthroses.

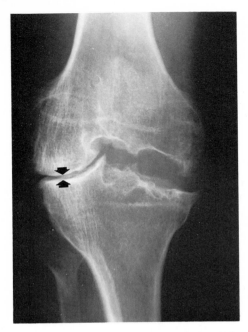

Fig. 26.5 The knee of a 23 year old haemophiliac. The intercondylar notch is widened due to repeated haemorrhage at the insertion of the cruciate ligaments, and there is subchondral cyst formation medially in both tibia and femur. These findings are unique to haemophilia. Destruction of the cartilage has resulted in narrowing of the lateral compartment of the joint (arrows). (Dr David Lewall, King Faisal Specialist Hospital, Saudi Arabia.)

Clinical Features
Limitation of movement initially.
Later there are fixed flexion deformities, bony swelling, crepitation and muscle wasting.
Marked joint disorganisation sometimes occurs.

Radiology
Degenerative changes.
Prominent periarticular cysts.
In children, widening of the epiphyses.
Disorganised joints resemble neuropathic arthritis.

Haemoglobinopathies

Thrombotic episodes, occurring during crises and involving bone, periosteum and periarticular tissues, appear to be the principal mechanisms underlying rheumatic manifestations of sickle cell disease and other haemoglobinopathies.
Musculoskeletal problems include:
— dactylitis—periostitis of metacarpals, metatarsal and phalanges
— synovitis with effusions
— haemarthroses
— septic arthritis
— osteomyelitis
— bone infarcts
— aseptic necrosis.

Leukaemia

ACUTE LEUKAEMIA

A rheumatic presentation is not uncommon especially in children who are sometimes initially misdiagnosed as having juvenile chronic arthritis.
Manifestations include:
— bone pain and tenderness
— polyarthralgia, sometimes migratory
— mono- or polyarthritis with effusions.
Symptoms are usually due to leukaemic infiltration into juxta-articular bone, synovium or the periosteum.
X-ray changes include:
— juxta-epiphyseal lucent bands
— periosteal elevation.

CHRONIC LEUKAEMIA

Joint disease is less common and usually occurs late.
Diagnostic confusion may be increased because:
1 rheumatoid factor and ANA may be positive.
2 serum uric acid sometimes elevated.

Malignant Lymphoma

Skeletal involvement may result in:
— bone pain
— pathological fracture
— synovial infiltration and arthritis.
There is an increased frequency of lymphoma in primary sicca syndrome.

Myeloma

Back pain:
— one of the most common presentations of myeloma
— due to marrow infiltration, osteopenia and vertebral collapse.
Amyloid arthropathy:
— rare.

HERITABLE, DEVELOPMENTAL AND STORAGE DISEASES

Many of the heritable, developmental and storage diseases are associated with skeletal abnormalities which could cause rheumatic problems, e.g.
Inherited disorders of collagen and elastin:
— Marfan's syndrome
— Pseudoxanthoma elasticum
— Ehlers-Danlos syndrome.
Mucopolysaccharidoses
Storage diseases:
— Gaucher's disease: sphingolipid storage abnormality
— Fabry's disease: glycolipid storage disorder.
Miscellaneous inherited conditions:
— epiphyseal dysplasias
— achrondroplasia.

Hypermobility Syndrome

Hypermobility is a feature of several hereditary disorders such as Marfan's syndrome and Ehlers-Danlos syndrome.
Normal individuals show considerable variation in joint mobility

but adults are considered hypermobile when they can:
— extend the fifth MCP joint $> 90°$
— appose thumb to volar surface of forearm
— hyperextend elbow and knee by $> 10°$
— place hands flat on the floor with knees extended.
Clinical manifestations may be minimal but include:
— susceptibility to joint trauma and dislocation
— joint effusions especially knee
— chronic low back pain
— premature osteoarthritis.

IMMUNOLOGICAL DISEASES

Hypogammaglobulinaemia

Primary hypo- and agammaglobulinaemia may be congenital or acquired.
10–30% of patients develop a chronic arthritis in which major features are:
— polyarticular, often symmetrical involvement of knees, ankles, wrists and fingers
— occasional nodules
— absence of rheumatoid factor
— absence of plasma cells from synovium which otherwise resembles rheumatoid arthritis
— non-erosive course
— response to gammaglobulin therapy.
Other features may include:
— recurrent infections
— lymphadenopathy, splenomegaly
— watery diarrhoea
— other connective tissue disease
— lymphoma.
Although the arthritis of hypogammaglobulinaemia was once considered RA-like, its features are more those of a reactive seronegative arthritis.

Serum Sickness

In acute serum sickness, a large antigenic stimulus produces an antibody response which, at a critical time of antigen excess,

results in immune complex formation and the development of:
— vasculitis
— arthritis
— glomerulonephritis.
A number of antigens, particularly animal proteins, can produce this response and such a mechanism is responsible for some drug reactions.

METABOLIC DISEASES

Haemochromatosis

Two types of arthritis may occur:
1 Haemochromatotic arthropathy, a peculiar chronic degenerative arthritis particularly affecting the second and third MCP joints.
2 Calcium pyrophosphate arthropathy, sometimes with episodes of acute synovitis.
Control of iron overload by venesection does not influence joint disease.

Ochronosis

The rheumatic manifestations are:

Ochronotic arthropathy:
— degenerative arthritis sometimes complicated by osteochondritis
— affects large joints especially knees.
Ochronotic spondylosis:
— low back pain and stiffness and limitation may resemble ankylosing spondylitis
— radiologically, occurs in and around multiple intervertebral discs with subsequent degenerative changes
— the sacroiliac joints are not involved.

Hyperlipoproteinaemia

A number of types of hyperlipoproteinaemia have been described and most may be associated with rheumatic problems (Table 26.1).

Table 26.1   Types of hyperlipoproteinaemia associated with rheumatic problems.

Type	Lipoprotein (LP) Abnormality	Rheumatic manifestations
II	Beta LP ↑ cholesterol	Tendon xanthomata Acute polyarthritis —migratory
III	Abnormal beta prebeta protein ↑ cholesterol ↑ triglycerides	Tendon xanthomata Hyperuricaemia
IV	Prebeta LP ↑ triglycerides	Arthralgia Arthritis Hyperuricaemia
V	Chylomicrons Prebeta LP ↑ cholesterol ↑ triglycerides	Hyperuricaemia

METABOLIC BONE DISEASES

Osteoporosis

In osteoporosis there is reduction of bone mass per unit volume with normal bone structure and mineralisation. It may be generalised or localised.

Generalised osteoporosis may be:

Primary
— associated with ageing
— senile, postmenopausal.

Secondary to:
— endocrine disorders, e.g. Cushing's syndrome, hypogonadism, etc.
— chronic diseases: alcoholism, malabsorption, malignancy, myeloma, rheumatoid arthritis, etc.

Iatrogenic:
— immobilisation
— corticosteroid administration
— heparin through chronic usage.

Rheumatic manifestations relate to bone collapse and fractures in the spine:
— back pain with or without symptoms of nerve root compression
— progressive thoracic kyphosis: 'widow's hump'.

Osteomalacia

Osteomalacic bone is qualitatively abnormal with inadequate mineralisation of osteoid (Fig. 26.6A).

In adults, the disease is called osteomalacia; in children, it is called rickets.

May occur as a result of:

Vitamin D deficiency
— decreased production due to inadequate exposure to sunlight
— decreased intake due to dietary deficiency
— decreased absorption due to malabsorption of fat
— decreased availability due to drugs, e.g. epanutin
— impaired liver hydroxylation due to cirrhosis
— impaired renal hydroxylation due to chronic renal failure.

Phosphate deficiency
Increased phosphate loss due to renal tubular defects, acidosis, etc.

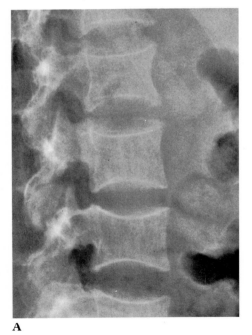

A

Fig. 26.6A   Osteomalacia in a 35 year old woman. There is deficient mineralization of osteoid and the soft vertebral bodies have been deformed by the intervertebral discs. (Dr David Lewall, King Faisal Specialist Hospital, Saudi Arabia.)

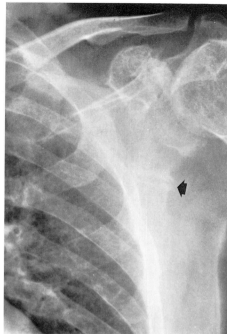

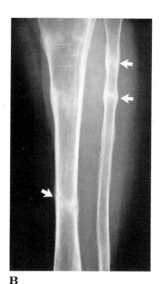

B   **C**

Fig. 26.6B Looser's zones in the tibia and fibule (arrows). These probably represent infractions with attempted healing. **C** Looser's zone in the scapula (arrows). (Dr David Lewall, King Faisal Specialist Hospital, Saudi Arabia.)

Decreased phosphate absorption due to antacids and malabsorption.

Rheumatic manifestations include:
— bone pain
  generalised ill-defined aches and pains, often without signs and commonly initially considered of psychological origin
— muscle weakness due to myopathy
— tetany.

Radiological changes (Fig. 26.6B & C) occur late and include:
— osteoporosis
— pseudofractures (Looser's zones)
and when renal failure is present:
— hyperparathyroid bone changes
— ectopic calcification.

Hyperparathyroidism

(*See* p. 275)

Paget's Disease

(*See* Chapter 22)

NEUROLOGICAL DISEASES

Neuropathic arthropathy (Charcot joint)

Loss or alteration of pain perception renders the joint liable to recurrent trauma and the development of severe and progressive degenerative changes with marked hypertrophic ostophyte formation.

Neurological disorders of the spinal cord and peripheral nerves which may cause neurogenic arthritis include:
— tabes dorsalis
— diabetes
— syringomyelia
— myelomeningocoele
— congenital indifference to pain
— peripheral neuropathies, etc.

CLINICAL FEATURES

Clinical features are:
— joint swelling and deformity usually, but not always, relatively painless
— bony swelling due to loose bodies, periarticular calcification and gross osteophyte formation
— joint effusions
— instability and sometimes hypermobility
— crepitus
— ultimately the joint may feel 'like a bag of bones'.

COMPLICATIONS

Complications include:
— fractures
— joint subluxation or dislocation
— infections of joints and bones.

RADIOLOGY

X-ray changes:
— marked degenerative changes

— destruction of bone ends
— massive osteophytes, periarticular calcification and loose
bodies.

RENAL DISEASES

Chronic renal failure

Chronic renal failure may be associated with:
Hyperuricaemia, but gout is uncommon.
Calcium pyrophosphate arthropathy, due to secondary hyperparathyroidism.
Renal osteodystrophy, a complex mixture of:
— osteomalacia
— hyperparathyroid bone disease.

Chronic dialysis

Chronic dialysis may be complicated by:
Periarticular calcification:
— calcium apatite deposition in periarticular tissues
— may provoke an acute inflammatory reaction.
Problems associated with chronic renal failure.

Renal transplantation

Renal transplantation may be complicated by:
Aseptic necrosis, due to high dose steroids.
Problems associated with chronic renal failure and dialysis.

RESPIRATORY DISEASES

Hypertrophic Pulmonary Osteoarthropathy (HPOA)

Also termed hypertrophic osteoarthropathy.
Most commonly associated with carcinoma of the lung but can be
classified as follows:
Primary:
— familial.
Secondary:
Intrathoracic neoplasm:
— bronchial carcinoma
— other lung, pleural or mediastinal tumours.

Suppurative pulmonary disease:
— bronchiectasis
— empyema and lung abscess
— tuberculosis.
Congenital cyanotic heart disease.
Inflammatory bowel disease.
Cirrhosis.
Graves' disease—thyroid acropachy.

CLINICAL FEATURES

Finger clubbing.
Painful swelling proximal to and around wrists, knees and ankles.
Joint effusions occasionally.

RADIOLOGY

X-rays are characteristic with periostitis along distal ends of shafts of long bones (Fig. 26.7).

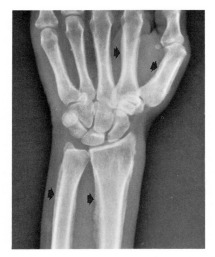

Fig. 26.7 Hypertophic pulmonary osteoarthropathy. This patient had a carcinoma of the oesophagus which eroded into the right lung resulting in an abscess. There is new bone formation along the radius, ulna and metacarpals (arrows). Many patients with this syndrome who have clubbing and bone pain do not have these radiological changes. (Dr David Lewell, King Faisal Specialist Hospital, Saudi Arabia.)

Fibrosing Alveolitis

Of patients with pulmonary fibrosis: >30% have positive rheumatoid factor and >5% go on to develop rheumatoid arthritis. Rheumatoid arthritis and pulmonary fibrosis are not thought to be causally related but since they occur together more often than expected, it is assumed that they share a common aetiological factor.

MISCELLANEOUS

Erythema Nodosum

May occur with a variety of underlying disorders including:
— sarcoidosis
— inflammatory bowel disease
— infections—TB, streptococci.
Arthropathy occurs in 50–75% of patients:
— arthralgia, arthritis or periarthritis
— occasionally precedes skin lesions
— involves ankles and knees, occasionally wrists and small joints
— remits spontaneously over weeks or months.

Sarcoidosis

Musculoskeletal manifestations include:
1 Erythema nodosum with arthropathy and bilateral hilar lymphadenopathy i.e. Lofgren's syndrome:
— a very common presentation of sarcoidosis
— fever may occur
— other manifestations of sarcoid typically absent.
2 Chronic sarcoid arthropathy:
— sarcoid infiltrates synovium
— usually non-erosive.
3 Bone involvement:
— cystic changes may occur in phalanges.
4 Myopathy:
— uncommon.

Amyloidosis

Amyloidosis relates to rheumatic diseases in two ways:
1 Chronic inflammatory diseases, such as rheumatoid arthritis

or juvenile chronic arthritis predisposes to the development of amyloidosis in a small number of patients:
— proteinuria is the usual presentation
— prognosis is poor.
2 Amyloid arthropathy (a rare disease):
— occurs almost exclusively in amyloid complicating myeloma; very rarely in primary amyloidosis
— may closely resemble nodular rheumatoid arthritis, e.g. symmetrical polyarthritis with prominent early morning stiffness; affects shoulders, small joints and knees particularly and elbow nodules show amyloid on biopsy.

Familial Mediterranean fever

Familial Mediterranean fever is an hereditary disease affecting particularly Anatolian Turks, Armenians, Leventine Arabs and Sephardic Jews and is characterised by amyloidosis and by recurrent attacks of:
— fever
— serositis of peritoneum and pleura causing abdominal and chest pain
— arthritis
    mono- or occasionally oligoarticular
    usually severe at onset
    lasting days or sometimes up to a year in the hip and knee
    protracted disease causes degenerative changes.

Non-metastatic malignancy

In addition to the rheumatic manifestations of malignant blood disorders, there are several entities reported in association with non-metastatic malignancy:
— hypertrophic pulmonary osteoarthropathy
— hyperuricaemia and secondary gout
— dermatomyositis and polymyositis
— carcinoma arthritis
    probably a valid entity since tumour removal sometimes induces remission of arthritis
    a rheumatoid-like inflammatory polyarthritis
    onset usually occurs before malignancy is recognised.

Index